Important Contact Information

NICU: _____

Nurse: _____

Other: _____

_____

_____

_____

_____

_____

_____

**Checking on Your Baby When You Are Not at the
Neonatal Intensive Care Unit (NICU):**
One very important piece of information for parents is the NICU phone
number, which you can call any time, day or night. If the nursery staff
are very busy or going through a shift change, they might have to
call you back. Some NICUs contact parents in other ways.
Ask the NICU staff about other options.

How to Use This Journal

Many families feel overwhelmed by the whole neonatal intensive care unit (NICU) experience. The *NICU Journal* was created to help them understand more about the NICU, record their baby's NICU events and achievements, and prepare for and celebrate the day when they take their baby home. It is formatted in such a way to help identify common issues and questions at each stage of the NICU stay, offer some tips on coping, and provide checklists to help track the baby's progress.

For ease of reading, we have used the pronoun "he" to describe a baby. Even though we are writing about singletons in most instances, the information provided is also applicable to multiples. Also, please check the glossary at the back of the journal to find definitions of terms that are commonly used in the NICU.

Parents are an important part of the baby's health care team. They have special qualities that no doctor or nurse can match, such as an intense love and distinct closeness, which their baby recognizes and finds calming. We hope this journal offers support, guidance, and comfort as you record your baby's NICU journey.

Best wishes from all of us at the Preemie Health Coalition.

Robin Bissinger, PhD, APRN, NNP-BC

Table of Contents

NICU Journal: An Introduction

Parenting in the NICU

Every baby is a precious gift. The neonatal intensive care unit (NICU) provides the medical care for those who are born too soon or are sick. When in the NICU, a parent's emotions can range from the joy felt over the birth of the baby and the progress being made to sadness or fear that naturally occurs when any baby is sick. Feeling overwhelmed as a parent in the face of unfamiliar situations is just another natural emotion that most parents of premature and sick babies feel.

Premature and sick babies might not be able to handle much holding or touching at first, and they might not like loud noises or bright lights, but babies do know the voice and touch of their parents, which helps in the baby's recovery and growth.

Getting to Know the NICU Staff

The NICU doctors and nurses are there to support not only the baby but the family as well. Staff will answer questions about the baby's condition and progress, and explain how the NICU works and what treatments may be needed during a hospital stay. A steady exchange of information is welcomed so that parents will make the best decisions for their baby in the easiest way possible.

About This Journal

The *NICU Journal* keeps track of important medical information, baby's NICU milestones, and memories of baby's early days. Hopefully, it will also serve as a guide to the entire NICU experience, with pages that help parents understand special health needs and ways for parents to help care for their newborn. Just as important, we have provided a place for you to write about this experience on a weekly basis. Other pages focus on how families can take care of themselves during this special, but difficult time. Each and every NICU situation is unique, and some of the sections in this journal may not be required reading for every family. Take what you need and leave the rest. You are not alone on this journey!

Your Baby's Arrival in the NICU

Parents can help care for their baby in the NICU from the very beginning, and this checklist is a good place to start.

- Talk to the nurses and doctors about your baby's schedule and when rounds occur.
- Ask if you can be there during medical and nursing rounds.
- Ask for a copy of the times that you are allowed to be with your baby.
- Give your contact information to the NICU staff (home, cell, and work telephone numbers).
- Talk with the NICU staff about how you like to learn (audio, visual, written).
- If you plan to breastfeed your baby, talk to a lactation consultant or nurse.
- Find a pediatrician. This will be your baby's main doctor after he leaves the hospital.
- Find out if the hospital offers any family support programs like parent mentors, breastfeeding support, or pumping groups.

NOTES:

Birth Experience

A place for the mother to record her memories of the birth experience.

Baby's Name:_____

The date I checked in was_____

You were born on _____ at _____ am/pm

Your actual due date was:_____

The hospital where you were born was:_____

The doctor who delivered you was: _____

About the birth:_____

_____

_____

_____

_____

_____

_____

_____

_____

Baby Arrival

A place to record memories of the baby's arrival.

Your eyes were _____ and your hair was_____

Your weight was _____ and your length was_____

Your doctor first said these words about you _____

_____

_____

Your stay in the NICU began on:_____

The name we chose for you:_____

Its special meaning: _____

_____

Thoughts and first impressions of you: _____

_____

_____

_____

_____

_____

_____

_____

Special Moments

During your baby's stay in the NICU, you will celebrate "firsts" and share many special experiences. Record these memories below so that you can always recall these joyful moments.

The first time...

I saw you up close: _____

I felt your skin: _____

You began to suck: _____

You wrapped your little fingers around mine: _____

We spent time together as a family: _____

You opened your eyes: _____

We did skin-to-skin (kangaroo) care: _____

You breathed on your own: _____

I held you in my arms: _____

You looked at me: _____

I saw you without equipment: _____

You cried out loud: _____

The first time I fed you: _____

You had a bath: _____

You wore clothes: _____

You moved to an open crib: _____

Other special moments you shared with your newborn in the NICU: _____

_____

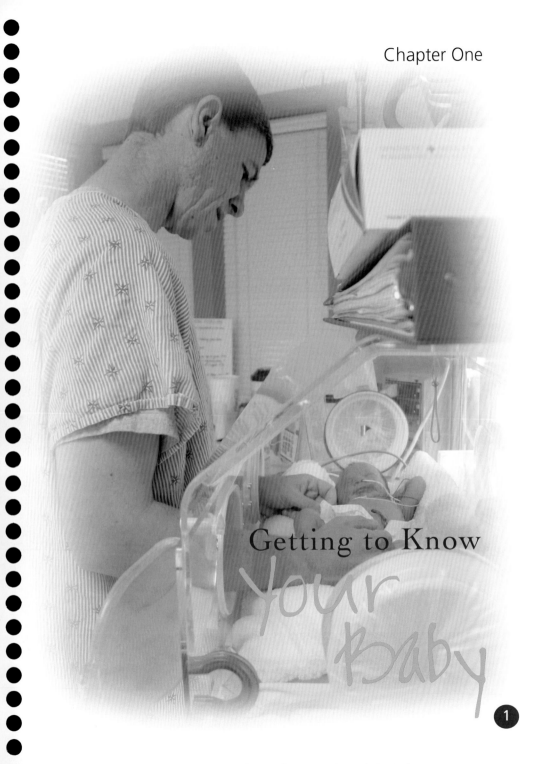

Getting to Know *Your Baby*

Your Baby's NICU Stay

During the NICU stay, parents learn how to care for their baby, including bathing, feeding, dressing, and holding the baby, as well as learning some routine medical care, such as taking a temperature.

You may feel nervous at first, but your baby's nurses will show you what to do. Taking care of your baby may help you feel a close connection. It also will help you feel more confident of your ability to take care of your baby after leaving the NICU.

As a parent, you can give unique and loving comfort to your baby. Medical technology is important, but your little one needs your gentle touch and nurturing voice. Just as your baby is so precious to you, you also are precious to your baby. It is helpful for you to learn the following:

- How to provide developmental care for your baby
- How to take baby's temperature
- How to care for baby's skin
- Identifying baby's special cues
- How to care for baby's cord area
- How to change a diaper
- How to give baby a bath
- How to do skin-to-skin (kangaroo) care
- Knowing the signs and symptoms of sickness
- Knowing your baby's diagnoses
- Knowing the plan for each of these diagnoses
- Knowing the medicines your baby needs and understanding side effects
- Understanding your baby's discharge equipment

Getting to Know Your Preemie

Any baby born early (less than 37 weeks of gestation) is considered premature. A premature baby's health can affect his growth and development. For example, health problems with the lungs, stomach, or brain may slow development. The following information will show how and when the senses and sleep and wake patterns develop, and how to tell if a baby is comfortable. It also gives advice on what you can do to let your baby know you're there.

Development of Your Baby's Senses
Our senses develop before we are born. The sense of touch starts during the first trimester of pregnancy. Taste, smell, and hearing begin during the second trimester. Babies usually do not begin to see until 40 weeks. Preemie babies, depending on how early they are born, may still need to develop these senses after birth.

How to Let Your Baby Know You Are There
Preemies are very sensitive to overstimulation. Try to focus on one of your baby's senses at a time. (For example, touch your baby and then talk to him—not both at the same time.)

CONCEPTION ⟶ 40 WEEKS

Touch

Smell and Taste

Hearing

Vision

| FIRST TRIMESTER | SECOND TRIMESTER | THIRD TRIMESTER |
| (0-13 weeks) | (13-26 weeks) | (26-40 weeks) |

Touch

Because babies develop this sense early, they are very sensitive to touch. Following these steps will help you use touch in a positive way:

- Use a constant, firm but gentle touch. A back-and-forth touch like stroking or massage can be too much for a premature baby.

- Gently cup one hand under the head and another hand on the bottoms of the feet to support a fetal position.

- Use skin-to-skin (kangaroo) care as soon as baby is ready. This can be comforting for both baby and parent.

- Put your finger in your baby's hand so he can hold it.

- Your baby will get used to your touch. Always touch your baby the same way each time you greet him.

Taste and Smell

Babies use taste and smell to know who their parents are while they are in the womb. They continue to use these senses to get to know you during the NICU stay as well.

- Do not wear perfumes or scented lotions.

- Place a pad that smells like your breast milk in your baby's isolette.

- Discuss with the doctor when to give the baby a pacifier that smells like your breast milk to suck during feeding times.

- Discuss with the doctor when to start nursing.

- When giving the baby a pacifier, you may need to hold it in his mouth. However, take it away if he does not seem to like it.

Hearing

Babies are able hear soft voices while they are in the womb. Talking to your baby after birth is another way for him to recognize you. The NICU is a loud place for babies, so try to avoid making unnecessary sounds.

- White-noise machines and playing music can make it harder for a baby to hear your voice.

- Keep other sounds (like closing drawers or scraping chairs) to a minimum when at the baby's bedside so your voice can be heard.

- Talk, read, or sing softly to your baby.

- Ask the nurses to help you recognize when even the sound of your voice might be too much for him.

Vision

This is the last sense to develop, so it needs the most protection. Very premature babies' eyelids may still be sealed closed at birth, but will open slowly over time. Even older babies usually need to be awake and calm for a while before they will start to use their eyes.

- Protect your baby's eyes by keeping the lights dim, covering the isolette with a blanket, and shielding his eyes from bright lights with your hands or a blanket during interaction.

- Visual stimuli, such as photos, should not be used until your baby is able to stay awake for longer periods of time.

- When your baby's eyes are open, keep visual stimulation simple. Your face is enough. Avoid adding more stimulation through voice or rocking when your baby's eyes are open.

- Toys placed in the baby's crib, while in the NICU, may be a potential source of infection. It's best to ask for permission from the health care team before adding a toy, stuffed animal, or other item to your baby's environment.

Preemie Gifts

During their first weeks or months of life, premature babies continue to develop as if they were in their mother's womb. Because of this, premature babies have special early growth experiences. Take time to celebrate these experiences as gifts that only premature babies have.

Sounds
Beginning at 33 weeks' gestation, babies make a sweet noise, similar to the sound a little lamb makes. This special sound usually lasts about 5 or 6 weeks. Record your thoughts and memories below.

_____

_____

Ears
At first, your baby's ears will lie close to his head. As he gets closer to the due date, the ears begin to extend and grow. Record your memories.

_____

_____

Fingernails
At first, the baby might have tiny fingernails—or even just nailbeds. During the first few weeks, watch closely as the nails begin to grow. Write your memories below.

_____

_____

Eyelashes
A baby's eyelashes may take a few weeks to grow. As you begin to see your baby's eyelashes, take time to remember this special gift below.

_____

_____

Footprints/Handprints

Each baby's handprints and footprints are beautiful. Each month leading up to the baby's actual due date, more lines will fill in the handprints and footprints. You may wish to ask a nurse to help take an imprint of your baby's handprints and footprints below.

Development of Your Baby's Sleep/Wake Cycle

Preemies and sick babies sleep most of the time. It is best to avoid waking them because they need sleep to grow and recover. As babies get closer to term age and get stronger, they will be able to stay awake for longer periods of time. Babies with health problems may not be able to increase their awake times until after their actual due date (around when we expected the birth to occur) or when they get stronger.

Signs that a preemie may be struggling with waking and staying alert.

- It is hard to tell if your baby is awake or asleep. He may move around a lot and open his eyes for short periods. His eyes may move around in his head. His breathing is irregular and he frequently twitches and startles.

- He may wake up suddenly with a start.

- He seems fussy with no clear awake and calm periods.

- When he is awake and calm, his eyes may seem glazed or dull. He may seem panicked or worried.

- When awake and calm, he may open his eyes very wide so that they look like they are popping out. He may stare at an object and not seem to be able to look away.

- When he is awake and upset, his cry is weak and strained, not rhythmic and robust.

- He may have trouble getting to sleep and staying asleep.

Signs that a baby's awake time is becoming more stable include the following:

- You can tell the difference between a light sleep and a deep sleep. During light sleep, your baby may twitch, startle, move his eyes under closed lids, and breathe irregularly, but he is clearly asleep. During deep sleep, your baby's breathing is regular, his eyes are still, and there is little movement.

- Your baby wakes up slowly with a drowsy period and his eyes open and shut over and over.

- You can tell the difference between your baby's sleeping and waking times. When he is awake, he is calm. His eyes are bright and focused and he may use eye contact to let you know he is ready to interact.

- Your baby has a strong cry.

- Your baby can calm himself by sucking on his fist or a pacifier, or by hearing your voice.

Developmental Care for Your Premature Baby

As a preemie, your baby needs special care and attention. Bright lights and loud noises may bother your baby, especially if he is very premature. You also may find that your baby needs to be held or positioned in certain ways. Learning the best way to care for your baby now can help him grow and develop down the road.

Lights and Sounds

Your premature baby needs calm surroundings. You can help the NICU staff create a comfortable space for your baby by protecting your baby's eyes from bright lights. If possible, lower the lights in your baby's room. You also should avoid making loud noises around your baby, and always try to speak softly to your baby.

Positioning and Holding Your Baby

It is important to provide your newborn with extra support when you are positioning or holding him. Your baby's NICU staff can teach you the most calming and supportive positions to place your baby. For instance, you can offer comfort and support to your baby by cradling your baby's head, bottom, or feet. These positions help your baby breathe well and help your baby's muscles develop properly. Proper positions also help your baby feel secure and lower his stress level.

Touch and Your Preemie

A premature baby's skin can be very fragile and sensitive to touch. Knowing what type of touch is best can help keep baby's skin healthy. The NICU staff will show you several ways to safely touch your baby, depending on your baby's age and size.

Constant, Steady Touch

Most preemies born at less than 26 weeks' gestation have very fragile skin and are very sensitive to touch. Don't be afraid to ask if it is okay to touch your baby. If it is not suggested at this particular time, ask when would be a good time. Once the medical staff has told you that your baby is stable enough to touch, hold your baby's hand or let your baby hold your finger. Do not stroke, rub, or pat your baby. Instead, touch your baby gently yet steadily in the same place. Ask how often and for how long would it be best for your baby to be touched and how you will know if he needs a break.

You also can cradle your baby's head, bottom, or feet at this age. Avoid moving or rocking as you cradle your baby.

Snuggling

Even though your baby needs special kinds of touch, there are ways you can snuggle with him. Surround your baby by placing your hands close to his face and holding his knees up to his chest in a relaxed, tucked position. You can snuggle with your baby in this way while he is resting or while he is receiving care. Snuggling can help your baby feel safe and secure.

Pain and Your Baby

If your baby shows any signs of discomfort, stop what you are doing and use your hands to cradle him in a fetal position. This is called facilitated tucking (or containment) and helps babies become calm. Babies also may use a pacifier to soothe themselves. Pay attention to how your baby reacts, since not all babies find this comforting.

Newborns receive special medical care and support in the NICU. However, some procedures, such as "heel sticks" (taking blood from the baby's heel), inserting intravenous (IV) lines, injections, and removing tape from the baby's skin, can be uncomfortable. Below are some tips on how to help ease your baby's pain and discomfort during these procedures.

How can I tell if my baby is in pain or uncomfortable?

Babies cry for many reasons–they want to be changed, fed, and held–so sometimes it is hard to tell if a baby is in pain. The NICU staff can help you learn how to tell if your baby is uncomfortable or in pain.

Signs of pain include the following:

- Changes in heart rate and breathing patterns
- Moving away or waving arms and legs
- Facial expressions
- Crying
- Changes in coloring and body stiffness

What can I do to make my baby more comfortable?

If your baby seems to be in pain, you can try the following to relieve him:

- Swaddling or rocking your baby
- Placing a small drop of sucrose (a sugar solution) or a few drops of your breast milk onto your baby's tongue
- Giving your baby a pacifier, either plain or dipped in sucrose or breast milk

- Touching your baby or providing skin-to-skin (kangaroo) care
- Keeping lights and noise levels down to create a calm environment
- Talking to your doctor about pain medicines for your baby

Hand Washing and Your Baby

Babies in the NICU are at risk for infections during their hospital stay. Premature babies are at more risk because of their immature immune system and their fragile skin. Hand washing is the most important way to protect a baby. Everyone should wash their hands before and after touching the baby. Wash your hands each time you enter the nursery and any time you have touched objects or items not located with your baby. Also wash your hands before and after you change your baby's diaper, or if you touch your face or blow your nose.

The NICU will have hand-washing areas with sinks, as well as alcohol-based product dispensers throughout the unit. Alcohol-based products (hand sanitizer or gel) are an alternative to hand washing with soap and water. We believe they kill more germs and are less drying to hands. The NICU staff will explain what the policy is for hand washing upon entry to the NICU and during your stay. Following is some important information.

Upon Entry to the NICU

- Remove any jewelry on your hands or wrists (you may leave a plain wedding band on).
- Place jewelry in your purse or pocket. If you cannot take your jewelry off, make sure you scrub carefully around the stones and under the bands.
- Scrub and clean for 3 minutes when you first enter the NICU.
- Wash every part of your hands using a rubbing motion.
- Wash over and between each of your fingers, then your wrist and then up to your elbows.
- Make sure your nails and nail beds are clean.

Hand Washing During Your Visit

If you already scrubbed or washed when you entered the NICU, you can wash or use an alcohol-based product (gel) to clean your hands during your time in the NICU.

Wash or use gel on your hands if you sneeze, cough, or blow your nose. Wash your hands before and after you change your baby's diaper.

Wash or use gel on your hands if you touch any area of your body that has a lot of germs (your nose, mouth, face, hair, shoes) or after going to the bathroom.

Wash or use gel on your hands between holding each baby if you have multiples.

If you are using soap and water, place the soap on your hands and rub your hands together making a good lather.

You must wash your hands for at least 30 seconds for germs to be killed.

If you use the alcohol-based product (gel) you should get enough gel to clean your hands for 15 seconds before it dries.

Other Important Facts

Germs love to hide under fingernails. Studies have shown that artificial nails increase the chance of infections. The NICU team has removed theirs and it is suggested that mothers of premature or sick babies do the same. If you do not want to remove your nails, then you should consider gloves when touching your baby during his hospital stay.

It is important to remember that your baby will need you and your family to continue hand washing even after going home.

Always speak out if you see anyone, even NICU staff, about to touch your baby without hand washing.

Changing Your Baby's Diaper

Babies need their diapers changed several times each day. Because this requires extra touching, your baby may find it stressful. Learning how to position and support your baby during diaper changes will help him stay calm and comfortable.

Getting Your Baby Ready for a Diaper Change

Start by gently cradling your baby's head or feet. This gentle touch can help soothe your baby. If your baby is younger than 33 weeks' gestation, place "boundaries," such as rolled blankets, around him. Support your baby's upper body by holding his arms close to his body, keeping the hands close to the face.

As your baby grows stronger, he may only need a pacifier to calm him during diaper changes. However, you might want to keep using the boundaries during diaper changes.

Changing Your Baby's Diaper

Gently remove the clothes and diaper on the lower part of your baby's body. Carefully clean the skin around the diaper area and slide the new diaper under your baby. Try not to lift your baby's hips or bottom off the table or put pressure on your baby's stomach.

Some preemies need to rest during a diaper change to help them stay calm. The NICU staff can help you look for clues that your baby needs to take a break during a diaper change.

Always remember to wash your hands before and after a diaper change to protect both you and your baby.

Skin-to-Skin (Kangaroo) Care

Skin-to-skin care (sometimes called kangaroo care) is a special way of holding a baby against a bare chest. Holding baby close will help parents feel more comfortable with their baby. The skin-to-skin contact also can improve the baby's health and development. Just ask if your baby is stable enough for you to provide skin-to-skin care. Once the medical staff has given you the go-ahead, take full advantage of this healing touch. Be sure to take note of this special moment.

What to Do

When your baby is ready for skin-to-skin care, undress the baby, leaving only the diaper in place. Unbutton your shirt and place your baby on your bare chest so that his chest and stomach are touching your body. Then place a blanket over his back. Remember that you should not wear perfume or smoke cigarettes (or have the residue of secondhand smoke on your clothing or in your hair) before skin-to-skin care with your baby.

Your baby may fall asleep. The NICU staff may want to monitor your baby during this time. Kangaroo care can last between 1 and 2 hours. This could be a perfect opportunity to take a photograph of your baby.

What are the benefits of skin-to-skin care?

Skin-to-skin care can help your baby

- Stay warm.
- Gain weight.
- Cry less.
- Keep heart rate, breathing, and temperature stable.
- Sleep better.
- Breastfeeding better.
- Move from an incubator to a crib sooner.

Skin-to-skin care can help you

- Increase your milk production (for mothers).
- Feel more confident about caring for your baby.
- Feel a special closeness with your baby.

Feeding Your Baby

Feeding your baby is a wonderful way to feel close to your baby. Breast milk is the best first food for your baby and helps protect against infections. We encourage all mothers to pump their breast milk, whether they wish to breastfeed their baby long-term or just while their baby is in the NICU. Not every mother is able to pump her breast milk, but, if you can, it is a great way to improve your baby's health and recovery.

Importance of Breast Milk

Breast milk provides many benefits for premature and sick babies. Breast milk is tailored by your body to meet the needs of the baby. It has more proteins, and these proteins are easier for the baby to digest. It also has a higher fat content and calories for growth. Babies who are breastfed have fewer infections because of the infection-fighting immunoglobulins found in breast milk. For premature babies, breast milk is even more important because of the premature intestines and kidneys. Babies who are breastfed do better, have a decreased risk of allergies, have improved eye and brain growth, and have better weight gain.

Pumping Breast Milk

Start pumping your breast milk as soon as you can after giving birth–within 6 hours if possible. This will help your body build up its milk supply. It also allows you to store your milk for your baby to use later. Your hospital will store your pumped breast milk for your baby in a safe area.

At first, try to pump every 2 to 3 hours, even at night. Try to reach a total of 100 minutes over an entire day. As your body builds up a milk supply, you may be able to reduce the number of times you need to pump each day. It is important to measure the amount of milk you produce each day. That way, you can be sure your milk supply is keeping up with your baby's needs.

Early Feedings

At first, your baby may need to be fed through an IV. But, once your baby is ready, he can be fed breast milk or formula through a small "gavage." This is a feeding tube that is inserted through the nose or mouth and goes to your baby's stomach. It can be used to feed your baby until he is ready for regular feedings by mouth.

Early feedings, often called "trophic" feedings, are provided to help your baby's intestines and prepare him for later feedings. It is important to provide breast milk for these trophic feeds if you can. Your baby only needs a few drops, often less than a teaspoon, during the first days. Remember, you can help with these early feedings. Talk to the NICU staff about how you can be involved.

Helping Your Baby Learn to Eat

Most premature babies need help learning how to suck, swallow, and breathe at the same time. You can help your baby strengthen his mouth muscles by giving him a pacifier or a clean finger to suck.

As your baby grows stronger and learns to suck, you can work with the NICU staff to start feeding your baby with a bottle. Your baby still will need help with sucking, swallowing, and breathing, so take this slow. Let your baby have a few sucks at the bottle and then let him rest and breathe for a few moments.

During these first feedings, your baby may get tired easily. Sometimes, you can help your baby eat longer by placing your finger under his chin and holding his cheeks lightly while he sucks on the bottle. Your baby's nurse can show you this technique.

Breastfeeding

Most premature babies cannot breastfeed right away. However, once you and your baby are ready, breastfeeding can be a wonderful experience, and you will feel good knowing that your breast milk is the best first food for your baby.

When your baby is ready, hold him to your bare chest and practice skin-to-skin (kangaroo) care. Your baby will be comforted by your closeness and your milk will flow more easily. When holding your baby skin-to-skin, practice guiding him to your nipple. In time, this may help your baby "latch on" to your breast more easily.

Each breastfeeding experience is different. It may take time to adjust to your baby's feeding style. For mothers of multiples, it is important to remember that, even if your babies are identical, they will be different from each other, and each breastfeeding experience is different from baby to baby and from feeding to feeding. A lactation consultant is available at most hospitals to help new mothers with breastfeeding.

Fortifying Breast Milk

Your baby may need the extra calories, protein, and minerals found in formula. If so, your baby's doctor may recommend that you add formula (or a breast milk fortifier) to your pumped breast milk.

Feeding Multiples

It is possible to breastfeed more than one baby at a time. If you decide to breastfeed your twins or triplets, here are some things you can do to make this a more positive experience:

- Work with a lactation consultant who has experience with multiples.

- Get as much sleep, food, and water as possible.

- Get tips, tricks, and suggestions from other mothers of multiples who have breastfed their babies.

- Have someone help position your babies when feeding 2 at a time—at least until your babies have enough neck support to move toward your breast on their own (usually until they weigh 10 lbs).

- Provide skin-to-skin care with your babies as much as possible.

- Pump your breasts after nursing to help increase your milk production.

- Encourage family members to learn about the benefits of breastfeeding premature multiples so that they can offer help and support.

If you are the mother of multiples, you should ask how best you can color code your pumped breast milk and how best to divide and store your breast milk from each pumping session, so that your baby who is healthiest and first ready to receive your breast milk will not be the only one to receive your very first and most beneficial early milk. Each of your babies, once they are ready to receive your milk, should be given your early expressed breast milk so that they will each be afforded the same benefits of this milk.

Bottle-feeding

If you decide not to breastfeed your baby or you are not medically able, you can still develop a special connection with your baby while bottle-feeding. To make the most of your time together, hold your baby close and look into his eyes during the feeding.

Bathing Your Baby

Preemies have delicate skin that requires gentle bathing styles, such as "spot" and "swaddled" bathing. Learning more about how to bathe your baby can help make it an even better experience for you both.

Spot Bathing

At first, a preemie may only need to be cleaned in certain areas, such as the mouth, diaper area, and around tubes or other equipment. Simply wet a soft, smooth cloth with clean water and gently wipe the spots on your baby that need cleaning, then dab the spots with a dry cloth.

If the NICU staff is bathing your baby, ask if you can hold your baby during the bath. You also can comfort your baby during bath time by offering a pacifier or holding his finger. It is not uncommon for a baby to cry the first few times he is bathed. This is a whole new experience and new sensation for him, and it will be important to be exceptionally gentle and slow in your movements and care.

Swaddled Bathing

As your baby grows stronger, he will be ready for a swaddled bath. Wrap your baby in a blanket or cloth. Next, place your baby in a tub of warm water so that the water touches the baby's shoulders. (Never let go during a bath.) Use a soft, smooth, wet cloth (without soap) to wash your baby's face by wiping from nose to ears. Once the face is clean, pat it dry.

After you have cleaned your baby's face, add cleansing lotion to your wet cloth. Remove one part of the blanket at a time to wash the body. Cover each area after you have washed it. Once you have washed your baby's entire body, use the soapy, wet cloth to wash the hair, then rinse the soap from your baby's hair with clean water.

Once you have finished bathing your baby, remove him from the wet blanket and wrap him in a warm, dry towel. Cover your baby's head to keep him warm and gently pat him dry. It is not uncommon for parents to feel clumsy or all thumbs the first few times they do this. This is a totally new experience for you, and your NICU staff knows this. They are there to help and support you as you learn to care for your baby.

Most first-time mothers of term babies do not have the gift of having a professional medical staff right at their fingertips to help them maneuver through this milestone—just another gift from your preemie or sick baby! Ask someone to take a picture of you and your baby during this big event, and don't forget to note this date on your Special Moments page.

Late-Preterm Infants

A baby born 3 to 6 weeks before his due date is often referred to as a "Late-Preterm" baby. Even though these babies are just slightly early, they are at risk to have their own unique medical and/or developmental problems. Even though a late-preterm baby may look very healthy, much like a baby born at full-term, he is at much greater risk for potentially serious health problems than full-term babies. Late preterm babies are also at higher risk for having to return to the hospital. If you have a late-preterm baby, here are a few things to pay attention to during the first year:

- While in the hospital and after discharge, your baby may take a little longer to feed and may need to eat more frequently. Work with the NICU staff to develop a feeding plan before you leave the hospital. It is very important that the baby takes in an adequate amount of breast milk or formula, especially in the first couple days of life when he is at greater risk for jaundice. Most mothers appreciate assistance from the lactation professional or nurse to help the baby latch on and maintain breastfeeding. Your baby may become tired and not nurse or bottle-feed very long. Ask your health care professional how many wet diapers a day your baby should have and how much your baby should eat.

- Initially, your baby may sleep longer than a full-term baby. It is important to make sure he eats at least every 4 hours. You may have to wake him for feedings if he is not eating frequently enough. Remember to put your baby on his back to sleep. Ask your health care professional how long your baby should sleep before you wake him.

- A baby's lungs are one of the last parts of his body to be fully developed and, even if your baby did not need additional oxygen or a respirator, your baby's lungs are still developing. Even though your baby was born just a few weeks before your due date, his lungs are immature and very sensitive. Secondhand tobacco smoke, perfumes, and environmental pollutants can irritate baby's airways and cause distress very easily. If your baby is having any trouble breathing, call 911 immediately and then call your baby's doctor. In advance, remember to ask your baby's doctor what the best way is to reach him or her.

Babies born early have less body fat than a term baby. This extra fat in the last few weeks of pregnancy is very important, and babies born even just a little early have more difficulty maintaining a normal body temperature and will lose heat very quickly. Cold, premature babies will use their calories to stay warm and will not grow and develop like they should. It is important to keep your baby away from drafts and keep the room warmer than you might otherwise. If you are going out in the colder weather or into air conditioning, consider using a hat and blanket to help keep the baby warm. Dress your baby in one layer more than you are wearing. Ask your health care professional how you can best assess the appropriate layer of clothing for your baby.

Your baby will be screened for jaundice before he goes home from the hospital, but he is still at risk for hyperbilirubinemia. Your baby will be tested for this just before discharge and you should find out the results of the hospital screening before you go home. Visit your pediatrician or primary health care professional within 24 to 48 hours after your baby comes home from the hospital. If your baby's skin appears yellow or orange in color and if he is not eating well, you should call his doctor immediately. Ask your baby's doctor or nurse how to best assess your baby for jaundice.

Like all newborns just leaving the hospital, your baby has not had all of his vaccines/immunizations, and you should be careful to avoid exposing him to people with infections. Avoid going out in crowds. Late-preterm babies have an immature immune system and are at a greater risk of infection than term babies. Watch for signs and symptoms of infection and call your pediatrician with any concerns. One of the best ways to avoid exposing your baby to harmful germs and viruses is through proper hand washing. Ask all visitors to wash their hands before touching your baby. Also ask visitors to postpone their visit if they are sick or have been around anyone else who is sick. Most people don't understand how fragile and vulnerable to infection preemie is, even when he reaches full term.

Caring for Preemie Multiples

Caring for more than one newborn in the NICU brings even more challenges. Each baby will have special needs and may act in different ways than his siblings. With twins or triplets, it is especially important to ask for help from family, friends, and NICU staff. This will allow the parents to spend precious time with each of their babies–getting to know them–and learning how to take care of them.

Caring for Multiples in the NICU

- To be sure that you get all the support you need for each baby, talk to the NICU staff about the following:
- Placing the babies close to one another in the NICU.
- Treating the babies as individuals rather than as a group, including keeping separate notes for each baby and ideally calling each by their first name instead of baby "A," "B," or "C."
- Color coding isolettes, bottles, and other equipment and supplies for each baby.
- Finding a lactation consultant who has worked with mothers of multiples.
- Finding support when you cannot be in the NICU because of work, other children at home, or your need for recovery time.
- Finding a support group for families with multiples.

When One of Your Babies Has Gone Home But One or More Remain in the NICU

Having one or more babies in the hospital while others are at home can be very sad and difficult for new parents. Some parents feel guilty for leaving their babies at home to spend time with the babies still at the hospital, or they may feel bad for leaving the hospital to spend time with the babies at home.

All these feelings are normal. Remember that you are doing everything you can to be with all of your children. In time, your babies will all be home and it will be easier to spend time together as a family. Check with the NICU staff to see if you are allowed to bring your other babies with you when you visit and check with your primary health care professional to see if it is safe for your newborn at home to return to a hospital environment for these visits.

Photographing Your Baby in the NICU

Many parents are reluctant to take a picture of their sick or fragile baby, but most appreciate the fact that they did, especially when they see their baby's growth and progress. Because of the special needs and environment of a baby in the NICU, following are some tips (developed by a professional photographer and mother of a former 27-weeks' gestation baby) for photographing your baby. We hope you will find it helpful to celebrate your baby's arrival and time in the NICU by taking photos, keeping journals, creating scrapbooks, or gathering other memories during this special journey.

Tip #1: Turn off the Flash.
Whether you are using a film, digital, or disposable camera, try to use natural light. The flash can scare a baby and interrupt the dark, quiet environment of the NICU. Soft window light is best, so take advantage of any windows in your baby's room. If you are taking pictures when it's dark, the overhead lights should be enough. If your baby is having phototherapy, the "bili" lights also will be enough.

Tip #2: Step Back or Get Close.
One unfortunate drawback to disposable cameras is that you cannot focus them, and pictures can easily get blurry. If you are using a camera that does not allow focusing, take a few steps back so that your photos are sharp. You can always crop them later.

On the flip side, if you have a camera that allows you to focus, don't be afraid to get close. Close-ups of your baby's face, feet, and hands are precious. You often can work around tubes, monitors, and other hospital equipment, though, in some instances, you might want to include these to remember how things were.

Tip #3: Think in Black and White.
Consider buying some black and white film, or, if you have a digital camera, convert your color photos into black and white. These photographs often have a more "timeless" quality to them. They also "soften" the image by downplaying the red skin, shiny equipment, and other items near your baby.

Tip #4: Put Your Baby in Context.

There always comes a time when parents cannot believe their baby was ever that small. When you photograph your baby, place an item nearby that puts his small size into context, like a wedding ring or your hand. (Remember to remove all items after photographing.) That way, you'll be able to see just how small your baby was. You can remind your child of that down the road ("I remember when I could slide daddy's wedding ring up your arm.").

Tip #5: Special Occasions You Might Want to Remember.

Having a baby in the NICU doesn't mean that you cannot celebrate milestones just like you would for a full-term, healthy baby. However, NICU milestones can be very different. So remember to take pictures when

- Your baby is weaned off the ventilator and moves to CPAP (see Glossary).

- Your baby doesn't have any tape on his face.

- Your baby breastfeeds or bottle-feeds for the first time.

- You "kangaroo" your baby for the first time.

- A sibling comes to visit for the first time.

- Your baby gets his first bath.

- Your baby moves from an incubator to a crib.

Tip #6: Don't Forget Your Baby's Caregivers.

The doctors and nurses in the NICU are committed to providing the best medical care for your baby. They also play an important role in caring for your family, and they form attachments to you and your baby. Take photos of your baby with special caregivers (the doctors, nurses, therapists, and social workers). All these caring individuals are a big part of your baby's first "friends."

Tip #7: Share Those Photos.

Friends and family are not always sure how to relate to a family with a baby in the NICU. By sharing photos and updates by e-mail or in person, you can provide more information about your baby and possibly ease their concerns. Once you leave the NICU, the staff loves to get updates and photos of NICU "graduates," so keep the photos coming! There are several secure Web sites that allow you to share your photos with your family and friends. One is called "Care Pages" (www.mostonline.org/CarePages) and the other is "Caringbridge" (www.caringbridge.org).

Tip #8: Don't Expect Perfection in Your Photos.

For many parents, it is just too overwhelming to take photos during this stressful time. If you like, leave a camera at your baby's bedside. Ask the nurses to take some photos until you feel up to the task. And don't be disappointed if your photos aren't perfect–you will still look back on them and they will stir up memories (good and bad).

While it is hard to believe right now, you will one day look back on these NICU photos and see just how far your baby has come. That is the greatest reward of all.

Journaling

Your Baby at _____ Weeks

Today's date is _____ and you are _____ weeks old.

You weigh _____ grams (_____ lbs, _____ oz), and you are _____ inches long.

Milestones you met this week:

_____

_____

_____

How we helped take care of you this week:

_____

_____

_____

_____

Things we learned about you:

_____

_____

_____

_____

Medications you are on this week:

_____   _____

_____   _____

_____   _____

Procedures and surgeries you had this week and the follow-up care you will need:

_____

_____

_____

Names of the doctors, nurses, and others who helped you this week:

_____   _____

_____   _____

Questions for the doctors, nurses, and others caring for you:

_____

_____

Other special thoughts and memories we had about you this week:

_____

_____

_____

Your Baby at ____ Weeks

Today's date is _____ and you are _____ weeks old.

You weigh _____ grams (_____ lbs, _____ oz), and you are _____ inches long.

Milestones you met this week:

_____

_____

_____

How we helped take care of you this week:

_____

_____

_____

_____

Things we learned about you:

_____

_____

_____

_____

Medications you are on this week:

_____   _____

_____   _____

_____   _____

Procedures and surgeries you had this week and the follow-up care
you will need:

_____

_____

_____

Names of the doctors, nurses, and others who helped you this week:

_____   _____

_____   _____

Questions for the doctors, nurses, and others caring for you:

_____

_____

Other special thoughts and memories we had about you this week:

_____

_____

_____

Your Baby at ____ Weeks

Today's date is _____ and you are _____ weeks old.

You weigh _____ grams (_____ lbs, _____ oz), and you are _____ inches long.

Milestones you met this week:

_____

_____

_____

How we helped take care of you this week:

_____

_____

_____

Things we learned about you:

_____

_____

_____

Medications you are on this week:

_____   _____

_____   _____

_____   _____

Procedures and surgeries you had this week and the follow-up care
you will need:

_____

_____

_____

Names of the doctors, nurses, and others who helped you this week:

_____   _____

_____   _____

Questions for the doctors, nurses, and others caring for you:

_____

_____

Other special thoughts and memories we had about you this week:

_____

_____

_____

Your Baby at ＿＿ Weeks

Today's date is ＿＿＿＿＿＿＿＿＿ and you are ＿＿＿＿ weeks old.

You weigh ＿＿ grams (＿ lbs, ＿ oz), and you are ＿＿ inches long.

Milestones you met this week:

＿＿＿＿＿＿＿＿＿＿＿＿＿＿＿＿＿＿＿＿＿＿＿＿＿＿＿＿＿＿

＿＿＿＿＿＿＿＿＿＿＿＿＿＿＿＿＿＿＿＿＿＿＿＿＿＿＿＿＿＿

＿＿＿＿＿＿＿＿＿＿＿＿＿＿＿＿＿＿＿＿＿＿＿＿＿＿＿＿＿＿

How we helped take care of you this week:

＿＿＿＿＿＿＿＿＿＿＿＿＿＿＿＿＿＿＿＿＿＿＿＿＿＿＿＿＿＿

＿＿＿＿＿＿＿＿＿＿＿＿＿＿＿＿＿＿＿＿＿＿＿＿＿＿＿＿＿＿

＿＿＿＿＿＿＿＿＿＿＿＿＿＿＿＿＿＿＿＿＿＿＿＿＿＿＿＿＿＿

Things we learned about you:

＿＿＿＿＿＿＿＿＿＿＿＿＿＿＿＿＿＿＿＿＿＿＿＿＿＿＿＿＿＿

＿＿＿＿＿＿＿＿＿＿＿＿＿＿＿＿＿＿＿＿＿＿＿＿＿＿＿＿＿＿

＿＿＿＿＿＿＿＿＿＿＿＿＿＿＿＿＿＿＿＿＿＿＿＿＿＿＿＿＿＿

Medications you are on this week:

_____   _____

_____   _____

_____   _____

Procedures and surgeries you had this week and the follow-up care
you will need:

_____

_____

_____

Names of the doctors, nurses, and others who helped you this week:

_____   _____

_____   _____

Questions for the doctors, nurses, and others caring for you:

_____

_____

Other special thoughts and memories we had about you this week:

_____

_____

_____

Your Baby at ____ Weeks

Today's date is _____ and you are _____ weeks old.

You weigh _____ grams (____ lbs, ____ oz), and you are ____ inches long.

Milestones you met this week:

_____

_____

_____

How we helped take care of you this week:

_____

_____

_____

Things we learned about you:

_____

_____

_____

Medications you are on this week:

_____   _____

_____   _____

_____   _____

Procedures and surgeries you had this week and the follow-up care
you will need:

_____

_____

_____

Names of the doctors, nurses, and others who helped you this week:

_____   _____

_____   _____

Questions for the doctors, nurses, and others caring for you:

_____

_____

Other special thoughts and memories we had about you this week:

_____

_____

_____

Your Baby at _____ Weeks

Today's date is _____ and you are _____ weeks old.

You weigh _____ grams (_____ lbs, _____ oz), and you are _____ inches long.

Milestones you met this week:

_____

_____

_____

How we helped take care of you this week:

_____

_____

_____

Things we learned about you:

_____

_____

_____

Medications you are on this week:

_____   _____

_____   _____

_____   _____

Procedures and surgeries you had this week and the follow-up care
you will need:

_____

_____

_____

Names of the doctors, nurses, and others who helped you this week:

_____   _____

_____   _____

Questions for the doctors, nurses, and others caring for you:

_____

_____

Other special thoughts and memories we had about you this week:

_____

_____

_____

Your Baby at _____ Weeks

Today's date is _____ and you are _____ weeks old.

You weigh _____ grams (_____ lbs, _____ oz), and you are _____ inches long.

Milestones you met this week:

_____

_____

_____

How we helped take care of you this week:

_____

_____

_____

Things we learned about you:

_____

_____

_____

Medications you are on this week:

_____   _____

_____   _____

_____   _____

Procedures and surgeries you had this week and the follow-up care
you will need:

_____

_____

_____

Names of the doctors, nurses, and others who helped you this week:

_____   _____

_____   _____

Questions for the doctors, nurses, and others caring for you:

_____

_____

Other special thoughts and memories we had about you this week:

_____

_____

_____

Your Baby at ＿＿＿ Weeks

Today's date is ＿＿＿＿＿＿＿＿＿＿ and you are ＿＿＿＿＿ weeks old.

You weigh ＿＿＿ grams (＿＿ lbs, ＿＿ oz), and you are ＿＿ inches long.

Milestones you met this week:

＿＿＿＿＿＿＿＿＿＿＿＿＿＿＿＿＿＿＿＿＿＿＿＿＿＿＿＿＿＿＿

＿＿＿＿＿＿＿＿＿＿＿＿＿＿＿＿＿＿＿＿＿＿＿＿＿＿＿＿＿＿＿

＿＿＿＿＿＿＿＿＿＿＿＿＿＿＿＿＿＿＿＿＿＿＿＿＿＿＿＿＿＿＿

How we helped take care of you this week:

＿＿＿＿＿＿＿＿＿＿＿＿＿＿＿＿＿＿＿＿＿＿＿＿＿＿＿＿＿＿＿

＿＿＿＿＿＿＿＿＿＿＿＿＿＿＿＿＿＿＿＿＿＿＿＿＿＿＿＿＿＿＿

＿＿＿＿＿＿＿＿＿＿＿＿＿＿＿＿＿＿＿＿＿＿＿＿＿＿＿＿＿＿＿

Things we learned about you:

＿＿＿＿＿＿＿＿＿＿＿＿＿＿＿＿＿＿＿＿＿＿＿＿＿＿＿＿＿＿＿

＿＿＿＿＿＿＿＿＿＿＿＿＿＿＿＿＿＿＿＿＿＿＿＿＿＿＿＿＿＿＿

＿＿＿＿＿＿＿＿＿＿＿＿＿＿＿＿＿＿＿＿＿＿＿＿＿＿＿＿＿＿＿

Medications you are on this week:

_____   _____

_____   _____

_____   _____

Procedures and surgeries you had this week and the follow-up care
you will need:

_____

_____

_____

Names of the doctors, nurses, and others who helped you this week:

_____   _____

_____   _____

Questions for the doctors, nurses, and others caring for you:

_____

_____

Other special thoughts and memories we had about you this week:

_____

_____

_____

Your Baby at _____ Weeks

Today's date is _____ and you are _____ weeks old.

You weigh _____ grams (_____ lbs, _____ oz), and you are _____ inches long.

Milestones you met this week:

_____

_____

_____

How we helped take care of you this week:

_____

_____

_____

Things we learned about you:

_____

_____

_____

Medications you are on this week:

_____   _____

_____   _____

_____   _____

Procedures and surgeries you had this week and the follow-up care
you will need:

_____

_____

_____

Names of the doctors, nurses, and others who helped you this week:

_____   _____

_____   _____

Questions for the doctors, nurses, and others caring for you:

_____

_____

Other special thoughts and memories we had about you this week:

_____

_____

_____

Your Baby at _____ Weeks

Today's date is _____ and you are _____ weeks old.

You weigh _____ grams (_____ lbs, _____ oz), and you are _____ inches long.

Milestones you met this week:

_____

_____

_____

How we helped take care of you this week:

_____

_____

_____

Things we learned about you:

_____

_____

_____

Medications you are on this week:

_____   _____

_____   _____

_____   _____

Procedures and surgeries you had this week and the follow-up care
you will need:

_____

_____

_____

Names of the doctors, nurses, and others who helped you this week:

_____   _____

_____   _____

Questions for the doctors, nurses, and others caring for you:

_____

_____

Other special thoughts and memories we had about you this week:

_____

_____

_____

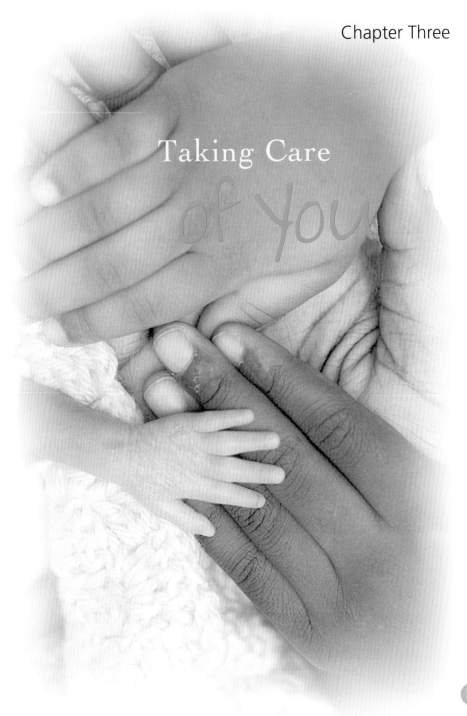

Taking Care
of You

Coping

Having a baby in a NICU is very stressful for parents. The uncertainty, the highs and lows, and the decisions all take their toll. If at first you feel distant from your baby, you may wonder if there is something wrong with you, or you may worry that because you cannot snuggle with your baby, you won't be able to bond.

Rest assured that feeling distant is a normal reaction for parents during the early weeks of their newborn's NICU stay. Feeling distant doesn't mean you are not bonding. Your bond with your baby began during pregnancy and continues to grow long after your baby is born. Be patient with yourself. Over time, as you adjust to the NICU, you'll feel closer and more like a parent to your baby.

As time passes and your emotions change, keep in mind that most parents of babies in the NICU feel many positive and negative feelings—even at the same time. This is because your heartfelt connection with your baby includes both joy and pain.

The NICU Roller Coaster:

For many families, the NICU stay is like a roller coaster ride, with ups and downs, triumphs, and setbacks. The following tips may help you deal with your baby's ups and downs:

- Give yourself permission to cry and feel overwhelmed. You may worry that you'll never be able to pull yourself back together, but you will.

- Get into a routine. Find a way to balance work, home, and visiting the hospital. Allow yourself to leave your baby's side when you can. While your baby needs you, it is also important to have time to yourself, with your partner, and with your other children. Also take time to do things you enjoy, like exercise. These restful breaks will help you find the strength to keep going.

- Connect with other parents of babies in the NICU. They share many of your feelings and struggles. Talk together, informally or in a support group. Ask the NICU staff if there are parents of babies who have graduated from the NICU with whom you can connect for support, or if there are other community resources.

- Explore your spiritual side. It might be helpful to reflect and lean on your spiritual beliefs. You may find comfort talking with a pastor, priest, rabbi, minister, or imam. It is normal for this experience to challenge your religious and spiritual beliefs. However, prayer, meditation, or quiet reflection can help you find emotional strength and hope during this challenging time.

- Keep a journal. Expressing your feelings on paper can help you cope with your emotional changes. A journal also strengthens your hope and patience, by reminding you how far you and your baby have come.

- Vent your frustrations. If your baby has a setback, you may be plunged back into fear and anxiety. Voice your fears, and hope for the best.

- Celebrate when you can. When your baby makes progress, it is okay to experience the joy.

- Accept the support of others, however clumsy it may seem. Let people know how they can best help you.

- Accept that you and your partner will react differently. Share your experiences and listen with empathy so that you each can feel supported.

You and Your Partner

During your baby's NICU stay, your partner can be your greatest source of support, but there may be times when you find it difficult to deal with each other. It's only natural that your reactions will be as unique as you are. The painful feelings so common to the NICU experience can add stress to your relationship. These tips may help you weather the crisis together:

- Share your thoughts, feelings, information, and burdensome tasks with each other. Lean on each other's strengths and forgive weaknesses. Remember that you both want what is best for your baby.

- Manage conflict with listening, compromise, and respect.

- Empathize with each other. When your partner is venting, don't try to fix it. Just listen and understand. Supporting each other is the best comfort.

- Make time to kindle and nurture your relationship, so that you can turn to it for strength.

Parents Without Partners in the NICU

If you are separated, divorced, single, or widowed, you may feel very alone without a partner to share the burdens and the joys. You may find it difficult to be the only one handling all the information and decisions. Being a single parent, you play a role that is challenging, but very important.

All parents need support. When you don't have a partner, it is natural to confide in a trusted family member or friend about your fears and concerns. Reach out to those close to you for the help you need. A NICU parent support group or other parents of babies in the NICU also can provide you with much needed comfort and partnership.

The March of Dimes (MOD) online community for NICU families (www.shareyourstory.org) offers support and information for families of babies in the NICU and who are home from the NICU. You can join in discussion with others who have very similar experiences to yours, ask questions, get support, participate in live online chats, and even offer your story and support to others.

Postpartum Depression

As a new mother, it is normal to have many intense feelings especially while your baby is in the NICU. It is not uncommon for new mothers to find that they may react differently or more passionately to some things than they may have prior to giving birth. This is completely normal. When do you know if what you are experiencing is something more than what would be expected for this time in your life? If you are having trouble dealing with the intense feelings, you may have some level of postpartum depression.

How do I know if I have postpartum depression?

If you have any of the following feelings, and cannot get rid of them, you may have postpartum depression:

- Sadness.
- Tiredness.
- Anger.
- Loss of hope.
- Loss of interest in things you like.
- Your ability to cope is not improving and you feel stuck.
- You find no joy in other parts of your life.
- You have trouble with your relationship with your partner or others close to you.
- You feel a parent support group isn't "quite enough."

It is essential to speak with a professional counselor if you
- Feel prolonged numbness or detachment.
- Continue to feel detached from your baby.
- Have trouble getting out of bed or starting your day.
- Feel unable to cope or manage your other responsibilities.
- Think about harming yourself or others.

A professional counselor can help. Your doctor or the hospital social worker can refer you to a counselor who understands the trauma of having a baby in the NICU. Even just a couple of visits might give you the reassurance and boost you need. Visiting a counselor and asking for help is nothing to be ashamed about; it will just help you cope better.

Content from www.marchofdimes.com, March of Dimes Foundation (2009). Reprinted with permission. For more information, go to www.marchofdimes.com or www.nacersano.org. To order materials, go to www.marchofdimes.com/catalog. For comfort, support and information from others who understand the challenges and uncertainties of the NICU experience, visit the March of Dimes' online community for NICU families, www.shareyourstory.org.

Smoking and Your Baby

It is very important for you to provide a smoke-free environment for your baby. Babies' lungs are not completely mature at birth and take 2 to 3 years to develop all the small air sacs necessary for a lifetime of healthy lung function. Tobacco smoke irritates the airways of babies and affects the growth of their lungs during the first 2 to 3 years of their lives, when their lungs are continuing to develop.

Premature babies are especially prone to having lung problems after discharge from the NICU. Being exposed to tobacco smoke makes these lung problems worse and makes premature babies more prone to develop airway infections and obstruction. When their parents smoke, premature babies smoke!

Many parents think that, as long as they smoke outside, their smoking does not harm their baby, but this is not true. Even when you smoke outside, chemicals from the tobacco smoke cling to your clothes and continue to irritate babies' airways, causing inflammation and airway injury. Anyone who smokes around a baby or young child is harming their precious child with secondhand smoke.

Secondhand smoke exposure has been well documented in many research studies to cause harm to babies and children. Babies exposed to secondhand smoke have increased upper and lower respiratory illnesses, increased ear infections, increased asthma, more frequent visits to the doctor, and more hospitalizations. Babies who are exposed to cigarette smoke have twice the occurrence of Sudden Infant Death Syndrome and are at increased risk for behavioral problems such as ADHD (Attention-Deficit/Hyperactivity Disorder).

The poisons from tobacco smoke cling to home furniture, drapes, carpets, ceilings, and walls, as well as car seats, for years. This is known as "thirdhand" smoke because it continues to "off gas" the toxic fumes for months to years later. It is important that you thoroughly clean your home and car when transforming them into smoke-free environments. A smoke-free home and car is essential for your baby to breathe safely.

Chemicals from tobacco smoke contaminate the breast milk that mothers produce. Breastfeeding is important for all babies to provide optimal nutrition and brain development as well as protection from infections. Because the protective benefits of breastfeeding are present even if a mother smokes, mothers who smoke are still encouraged to breastfeed their babies. If a mother who breastfeeds uses nicotine replacement therapy, this is much better for her baby than smoking. Of course, having no exposure to tobacco toxins is best for both mother and baby.

Babies and children who are exposed to secondhand smoke have much more serious health problems than babies or children who are not exposed to secondhand smoke. The consequences of using tobacco products is something we wish to help you avoid for both you and your baby.

Please let us know if you would like help in becoming a nonsmoker or if you have any questions about providing a smoke-free home and car for your baby. For the health of your baby and for your own health, it is essential that you and everyone in your household stop smoking.

Because tobacco products contain nicotine, which is very addictive, it is hard for most people to quit smoking. Fortunately, today there is help, which can make it easier to quit smoking, even if you have tried quitting before without success. This time you can succeed. Ask your pediatrician and call the quitline (1-800 QUIT-NOW) for help in quitting and in making your home and car smoke-free.

Journey
Home

Bringing Your Baby Home From the NICU

As baby grows stronger and healthier, the time will come to take him home. While some parents may feel excited, they also may worry about caring for the baby on their own. However, the NICU staff will work with families to make sure they know how to care for their baby on their own. Use this checklist as you prepare for going home.

Preparing for Your Baby to Leave the NICU

In the Hospital:

☐ Add your baby to your health insurance policy.

☐ Speak with a social worker to see if you qualify for state or local services and fill out the paperwork while your baby is still in the hospital.

☐ Request a predischarge meeting with your baby's health care team to talk about the baby's medical needs and what to expect in the months and years ahead.

☐ Choose a health care professional for your baby after discharge from the hospital, asking specific questions about his or her experience and any special care given for a premature or sick baby.

☐ If your baby is going to be on Medicaid and you are going to receive WIC, set it up while you are in the hospital.

Pediatric and Specialty Care

☐ Schedule your baby's first visit with the pediatrician.

☐ Schedule any follow-up appointments with specialists.

☐ Ask the NICU staff if your baby qualifies for an early intervention evaluation and have this scheduled before leaving the hospital.

☐ Make sure your baby has received all required immunizations (up to 2 months old).

☐ File your baby's immunization record in a folder for safekeeping and for upcoming health care visits.

☐ If your baby was born at or before 30 weeks' gestation, make sure your baby has an eye examination. Ask if you need to schedule a follow-up eye examination for your baby.

☐ Ask for the results of your baby's hearing screening. Also, ask if you need to schedule a follow-up visit for your baby.

☐ Get a copy of your baby's discharge summary for your records and be sure to review any and all questions about his care up until this point from your notes in your NICU Journal.

☐ Get all your baby's prescriptions from the doctors and review them with his health care team so that you are sure you understand how and when to administer any medications and have them filled.

☐ Make sure you know about Respiratory Syncytial Virus (RSV) season and what you need to do to protect your baby during the RSV season.

☐ Review the signs and symptoms of sickness that would make you call or visit your baby's pediatrician.

☐ Ask the NICU staff if you can stay in the NICU overnight ("room in") with your baby before discharge.

☐ Talk to the social worker if you are worried about electricity, phone service, transportation, or food when your baby leaves the NICU.

Safety

☐ Take a CPR (cardiopulmonary resuscitation) class.

☐ Get a car seat for your baby. Sometimes, premature babies have special needs because of their size and strength. They may need a car bed because of problems with apnea, oxygenation, and heart rate. Ask your care team what is best for your baby.

☐ Bring your baby's car seat to the hospital for a car seat test.

☐ Ask the NICU staff when your baby can safely go out in public.

☐ Discuss "back to sleep" and "tummy time" with your NICU staff.

Preparing for Your Baby's Medical Needs at Home

☐ Discuss with your care team any special medical supplies you will need in your home.

☐ Learn about any equipment your baby will need at home and who to call for additional questions.

☐ Learn how to order more equipment or supplies for your baby.

Preparing Your Home for Your Baby's Arrival

Preparing your home for your baby's arrival can help keep your baby healthy and safe. To prepare your home for your baby, you can

- ☐ Gather and store baby supplies, such as diapers, blankets, washcloths, formula, bottles (if you are not breastfeeding) and a digital (not mercury) thermometer.

- ☐ Prepare a crib for your baby or talk about other sleeping options for your baby with your health care professional.

- ☐ Post emergency phone numbers next to all the phones in your home.

- ☐ Clean your house of dust, pet hairs, paint smells, tobacco smoke, or other smells that may bother your baby's eyes, nose, and lungs.

- ☐ Teach everyone in your home about good hand washing. Be sure to have soap by all bathroom sinks. Having hand cleansers in any rooms in which you will take the baby is recommended.

Discuss with extended family and friends the precautions you will be taking to ensure continued good health of your preemie. Ask for their respect and support in doing so. Precautions, such as not allowing smoking in your home, asking anyone who may be "coming down with something" to postpone their visit, teaching everyone to do proper hand washing prior to touching the baby, limiting the number, and the length, of time you have guests (outside family included) and initially, the number of small children other than those who already live with you, to ideally reduce the possibility of exposure to illnesses especially during the cold season.

Preparing for Your Baby's Nutritional Needs at Home

- ☐ Discuss with your care team the special feeding needs of your baby at home.

- ☐ Take any stored breast milk home and review the care and thawing process for use at home.

- ☐ Babies who have been born prematurely may need to continue to receive additional nutrition after discharge with special formulas if they are not receiving human milk. This is to help these babies grow and improve outcomes. Those receiving human milk may also require a supplement.

☐ Consult your baby's doctor about whether any supplements are needed after discharge. These special formulas or breast milk supplements used after discharge may contain extra protein, calcium, phosphorous, vitamins, and minerals that promote adequate growth and provide energy. Again, your baby's health care professionals will determine which nutritional strategy to follow when you take your baby home and how to monitor your baby's growth and development.

Baby's Transportation Needs

All 50 states now have laws requiring the use of infant safety seats in the car, and it has become standard hospital policy that parents must have one in their possession before taking their new baby home. Showing up with a car safety seat, however, is not the same as using and installing it correctly. Make sure you use the installation tips provided by the manufacturer.

The "Car Seat Challenge"

For babies born more than 3 weeks prematurely, the American Academy of Pediatrics (AAP) recommends that they be monitored in their car seat before leaving the hospital. Taking this simple precaution helps ensure that the car seat's semi-reclined position won't cause the newborn to experience breathing problems or slowing of the heartbeat. When it is a problem, doctors may recommend that a baby use a car bed. Hospital staff who are trained in positioning babies properly in the car seat, and in detecting apnea, bradycardia, and oxygen desaturation, should conduct the car safety seat observation. Ask your health care team to review the car seat challenge with you and go over proper positioning for your baby.

Car safety seats ("regular" infant car seats) are recognized to provide excellent protection for babies positioned rear facing and are the preferred method of transportation. Car beds are meant for babies who cannot be safely restrained in a regular car seat and must be transported lying down. Most commonly, this applies to very small and/or premature babies. Car beds should never be bought secondhand or reused unless advised by a child passenger safety professional. Unlike car seats, most car beds are designed for one-baby use—even if only used for a few days or weeks.

The key to keeping your baby safe in the car lies not just in buying an appropriate car seat, but also in using it properly. Properly installed infant car seats have been shown to dramatically reduce the number of deaths (by some estimates, more than 70%) in children younger than 1 year.

A guide for families on car seat safety can be found at www.HealthyChildren.org.

Early Intervention Program

Preemie babies develop at their own pace and, along the way, they may need special Early Intervention services. Early Intervention is the official name for the extra care some children receive to help them develop, grow, and learn. An evaluation for Early Intervention services is available to your baby after discharge (anytime between birth and age 3 years) if he meets any of the following criteria:

- Your baby was admitted to the NICU or had a serious illness at birth that could affect the baby's development.
- Your baby was born with a low birth weight (less than 2,500 g) or born very premature (less than 33 weeks' gestation).
- Your baby was born with a birth abnormality that affects his brain, muscles, or nervous system.
- Your baby was exposed to alcohol or drugs before, during, or following your pregnancy.
- Your baby has been involved in a protective services case or program.

Ask your baby's NICU staff for information on how to set up an appointment for a free evaluation. Remember, you can ask for an evaluation even if you are not worried about your baby's progress or development. Qualifications can vary among states, so ask your health care professional about the Early Intervention Program (IEP) in your state.

When Your Baby Must Transfer Hospitals or Units

Transferring Your Baby to Another NICU

If your baby is very sick, he may need to go to a larger hospital or a regional medical center. These hospitals often have more specialists and resources to help babies with special health care needs. If your baby is moving to another hospital, talk to the hospital staff about how this will happen. Usually, your baby's current doctor will coordinate with the new NICU to help prepare your baby for traveling.

It may not be possible for you to travel with your baby. Ask the NICU staff about this. Make sure that you have the contact information for the new NICU so that you can call to check on your baby at any time.

Transferring Your Baby to an Intermediate Care Nursery

Very ill babies are cared for in the intensive care unit (ICU). As they begin to recover, they often go to an intermediate care nursery. This may be another unit in the hospital or at a different hospital.

The intermediate care nursery staff are trained to give the special medical attention babies need to grow stronger and more stable. If your baby is moving to an intermediate care nursery, talk to your doctor about how you can prepare for the change. For example, you may want to visit the new nursery and talk with the staff before your baby is transferred.

Your Baby's Health Maintenance and Immunization Records

Before discharge, your baby will receive the following:
- Immunizations
- An eye examination (if needed)
- A hearing screening
- Newborn screening blood spot tests
- Several doses of important medicines (if needed)

Keep a record of when your baby gets each of these, and note any follow-up you will need to do (when, where, and with whom, as well as the contact information, address, and directions to the office).

Immunizations
Immunizations protect your newborn from many infections. Below is a list of the ones your baby needs and a place for you to keep track of when your baby gets them. Preemies get their immunizations at the same age as full-term babies except for hepatitis B vaccine. Generally, no correction is made for being born early, and vaccinations are not delayed. It is very important that parents of preemies as well as those of all infants adhere to the recommended schedule for these immunizations. Some of these diseases have resurged in recent years in the United States, and babies who have been in the NICU are at increased risk for complications if they were exposed to them. It is equally important that the parents, siblings, and all caregivers are also immunized against pertussis (whooping cough) and influenza (flu). Premature babies are especially vulnerable to these infections that can cause severe lung infections and even death in young infants.

Hepatitis B
Hepatitis B is a serious disease that affects the liver. Hepatitis B vaccine prevents hepatitis B infection, and the serious consequences of hepatitis B virus infection, including liver cancer and cirrhosis. Three doses of the hepatitis B vaccine are safe and highly effective. The first shot is usually given before discharge from the hospital after birth to term and preterm babies who weigh more than 2 kg (4 lbs, 6 oz). The second shot is given between 1 and 4 months of age. The third shot is given between 6 and 18 months of age. If your baby's birth weight was less than 2 kg, 4 doses of hepatitis B vaccine are needed and the timing of the doses may vary. The doctor will tell you when shots will be given.

Your baby was given the hepatitis B vaccine on the following dates:

1st dose:_____

2nd dose:_____

3rd dose: _____

4th dose (if needed):_____

Follow-up needed after discharge:_____

_____

_____

Diphtheria, Tetanus, and Pertussis (DTaP)
The DTaP vaccine helps protect your baby from 3 diseases: diphtheria, tetanus, and pertussis (whooping cough). Three shots of the vaccine are needed within the first year of life. A fourth shot is given at 15 through 18 months. The fifth shot will be given at 4 through 6 years.

Your baby was given the DTaP vaccine on the following dates:

1st dose:_____

2nd dose:_____

3rd dose: _____

4th dose: _____

5th dose: _____

Follow-up needed after discharge:_____

_____

_____

Haemophilus influenzae type b

Haemophilus influenzae type b (Hib) is a type of bacteria that can cause several kinds of serious infections, including meningitis. Two or 3 shots of the Hib vaccine are needed within your baby's first 6 months of life. A booster dose is given at 12 to 15 months.

Your baby was given the Hib vaccine on the following dates:

1st dose:_____

2nd dose:_____

3rd dose:_____

Booster: _____

Follow-up needed after discharge:_____

_____

Polio

Three shots of the polio vaccine (also called inactivated polio vaccine, or IPV) are given between 2 and 18 months of age. A booster shot will be given when your child is between 4 and 6 years of age.

Your baby was given the polio vaccine on the following dates:

1st dose:_____

2nd dose:_____

3rd dose:_____

Booster: _____

Follow-up needed after discharge:_____

_____

Measles, Mumps, and Rubella (MMR)

The MMR vaccine will help protect your baby from measles, mumps, and rubella (German measles). The first shot is given when your child is between 12 and 15 months old. A second shot is usually given when your child is between 4 and 6 years of age but can be administered as early as 28 days after the first dose.

Your baby was given the MMR vaccine on the following dates:

1st dose:_____

2nd dose:_____

Follow-up needed after discharge:_____

Pneumococcal

Pneumococcus is a type of bacteria that can attack different parts of the body and cause serious infections. Three doses of this vaccine are given when your baby is 2, 4, and 6 months old. A fourth dose is given when your baby is between 12 and 15 months of age. If your baby is late getting these shots, check with your baby's doctor to see if fewer shots are needed and when your child should get them.

Your baby was given the pneumococcal vaccine on the following dates:

1st dose:_____

2nd dose:_____

3rd dose:_____

4th dose: _____

Follow-up needed after discharge:_____

Influenza (Flu)

The flu vaccine is given each year to all children between 6 months and 18 years of age. It is very important that if your baby is younger than 6 months that all family members and caregivers get the flu vaccine to protect the baby from catching the flu. Influenza infections in premature babies cause them to become critically ill. The first year that your baby receives the flu vaccine, he will get 2 shots separated by 4 weeks.

Your baby was given the flu vaccine on the following dates:

1st dose:_____

2nd dose *(4 weeks after the 1st dose):*_____

Follow-up needed after discharge:_____

_____

_____

Varicella (Chickenpox)

One dose of the chickenpox vaccine is given when your child is between 12 and 15 months old. A second shot is given when your child is 4 to 6 years of age, but it can be administered earlier.

Your baby was given the chickenpox vaccine on the following dates:

1st dose:_____

2nd dose:_____

Follow-up needed after discharge:_____

_____

_____

Other Immunizations

If your baby's doctor recommends other vaccines for your baby, record the dates she received the doses.

Your baby was given the vaccine on the following dates:

1st dose:_____

2nd dose:_____

3rd dose: _____

Follow-up needed after discharge:_____

_____

_____

Combination Vaccines

Your baby's doctor may combine vaccines to reduce the number of shots your baby needs to stay healthy. If you are interested in combining your baby's vaccines, check with your baby's doctor to see if any are available. Examples of common combination vaccines include the following:

- DTaP and Hib vaccine
- Hib and hepatitis B vaccine
- DTaP, hepatitis B, and polio vaccine
- MMR and varicella (chickenpox) vaccine

Note: Immunization information is updated periodically. Please go to www.HealthyChildren.org for the most current information.

Respiratory Syncytial Virus: More Than a Cold

Respiratory syncytial virus (RES-pri-tor-ee sin-SISH-shul VYE-ris), or RSV, is a very common illness in infancy and early childhood. Most infants get RSV during their first year of life, and almost all children are infected by the time they are 2 years old. For most healthy children, RSV is like a cold. However, for some preterm babies and for those with certain types of lung or heart problems, it can be dangerous. This is because premature babies, even those who did not need any additional help breathing while they were in the NICU, do not have fully developed lungs. Also, they may not have received virus-fighting substances (called antibodies) to help fight off RSV and other viruses. It is not uncommon for parents to feel that their once very tiny and fragile newborn now appears very healthy and robust, but it is still extremely important during this first year of life to take specific precautions to decrease exposure to RSV if at all possible. If your baby is younger than 1 year at the beginning of RSV season, you should take appropriate precautions, such as continued proper hand washing and limiting exposure to crowds and school-aged children. Speak with your baby's health care professional for additional suggestions.

RSV infections tend to occur at a certain time of the year. The season usually starts in the fall and ends in the spring. Talk with your child's doctor about the RSV season in your area. For babies born before 29 weeks' gestation or with certain other risk factors, you need to take special precautions to help ensure they are not exposed to a person with RSV or any other cold, flu, or virus. It is very important to be sure your child is not exposed to secondhand smoke. Breastfeeding will help protect your baby from many types of infection.

RSV is contagious. It can be spread through the air when a person coughs or sneezes. RSV also can spread by touching an object that has the virus on it. In fact, the virus can live on countertops, doorknobs, hands, and clothing for up to 7 hours. Hand washing and proper cleaning is the best way to help prevent the spread of RSV.

Symptoms of RSV
RSV usually causes a mild cold with a runny nose and fever. However, in some babies, the symptoms can become severe. Call your doctor right away if your baby has any of these symptoms:

- Cough that does not go away or gets worse
- Wheezing (a high-pitched whistling sound when breathing)
- Trouble breathing or breathing faster than usual
- Blue color on the lips or around the mouth
- High fever
- Thick nasal discharge

Eye and Ear Health

A baby's eye and ear health is very important, especially for a preemie. When your baby gets his eye examination and hearing screening, you can keep track of the results and the necessary follow-up care with a hearing or vision specialist.

You had your newborn eye examination on this date: _____

RESULTS:_____

_____

Follow-up needed after discharge:_____

_____

You had your newborn hearing screening on this date:_____

Left Ear: **Right Ear:**

☐ Passed   ☐ Passed

☐ Failed   ☐ Failed

Follow-up needed after discharge:_____

_____

_____

_____

_____

_____

Safe Sleep and Your Baby

Many infants die during sleep from unsafe sleep environments. Some of these deaths are from entrapment, suffocation, and strangulation. Some infants die from sudden infant death syndrome (SIDS), which is the sudden, unexplained death of a baby younger than 1 year. However, the following are ways for parents to keep their sleeping baby safe.

- Place your baby to sleep on his back for every sleep until he is 1 year old. If your baby has rolled onto his side or stomach, he can be left in that position if he is already able to roll from tummy to back and back to tummy. If your baby falls asleep in a car safety seat, stroller, swing, infant carrier, or infant sling he should be moved to a firm sleep surface as soon as possible.

- Place your baby to sleep on a firm sleep surface. The crib, bassinet, portable crib, or play yard should meet current safety standards. Do not put blankets or pillows between the mattress and the fitted sheet. Never put your baby to sleep on a chair, sofa, water bed, cushion, or sheepskin.

- Keep soft objects, loose bedding, or any objects that could increase the risk of entrapment, suffocation, or strangulation out of the crib. These objects include pillows, quilts, comforters, sheepskins, bumper pads, and stuffed toys. *Note:* Research has not shown us when it's 100% safe to have these objects in the crib; however, most experts agree that after 12 months of age these objects pose little health risk to healthy babies.

- Place your baby to sleep in the same room where you sleep but not the same bed. This is the safest sleep arrangement for your baby. Put your baby's crib close to your bed, so that you can easily watch and feed your baby.

- Breastfeed as much and for as long as you can.

- Make sure that your baby gets all recommended immunizations.

- Keep your baby away from smokers and places where people smoke.

- Do not let your baby get too hot. In general, dress your baby in no more than one extra layer than you would wear. Your baby may be too hot if she is sweating or if she feels hot. If you are worried that your baby is cold, you can use infant sleep clothing.

- Offer a pacifier at nap time and bedtime. This helps to reduce the risk of SIDS. If you are breastfeeding, wait until breastfeeding is going well before offering a pacifier. It's OK if your baby doesn't want to use a pacifier. If the baby's pacifier falls out after he falls asleep, you don't have to put it back in.

Note: These recommendations are for healthy babies up to 1 year of age. A very small number of babies with certain medical conditions may need to be placed to sleep on their stomachs. Your baby's doctor can tell you what is best for your baby.

Chapter Four

Supporting You
and Your Preemie

Milestone Guidelines for Premature Babies

Having a baby–whether it's your first child or your fourth– is so exciting! But it is not always easy. If your baby was born more than 3 weeks early, you may have more questions about your baby and how he will grow than a parent whose baby was born on time.

We wrote this section to help you understand how your child will develop. We have listed important milestones–or achievements–in a child's growth, so you know what to watch for at each age. For example, typical milestones for babies are, "makes eye contact and smiles" and "rolls from tummy onto back."

It is important to remember that development is not a race. Babies develop at their own speed and in their own way. Some children do not reach every milestone at the same time. *This is especially true if they were born early.*

Adjust your baby's age to get a true sense of where your baby should be in his development.

Here's what to do: If your baby is 14 weeks old, but was born 6 weeks early, subtract 6 from 14. This gives you 8 weeks. Use this adjusted age when you look at the milestones sections.

By age 2 years, most children have caught up to the normal range, and you won't have to do this math. If your child has not caught up, he may require extra support for a longer period of time.

Watch for progress. The most important thing is to make sure your child is moving forward in his development. For example, your baby should progress from pulling himself up, to standing, and then to walking. Remember that children reach new milestones at different ages.

You will know your child better than anyone else. When you watch him carefully, you will see ways he is growing well.

You also will know if he needs more help. Remember, you do not have to do it alone. There are doctors, teachers, and other people and information to support you. We hope this information gives you a good place to start.

A Guideline to the Milestones in a Child's Development

The following information shows how young children typically develop. It is important to use your child's adjusted age when tracking his development. So, if your baby is 21 weeks old, but was born 5 weeks early, his adjusted age is 16 weeks (or 4 months). This means you should refer to the milestones listed under "at 4 months (16 weeks)" to see what your child should be doing at this age.

Use this information to help you watch your child's progress.

At 2 months
(8 weeks)

Motor
- Moves hands and legs actively
- Keeps hands open most of the time
- Lifts head and chest when lying on tummy
- Controls head a little, but may still need support
- Holds objects in hands

Language
- Responds to sounds (for example, turns when hears voices and rattles)
- Makes cooing noises like "aaaah" and "ooooh"
- Cries when needs something

Activities
- Fixes eyes on a person or object (a mobile, for example) and follows its movement
- Has different cries for different needs

Social/Emotional
- Makes eye contact and smiles
- Recognizes and enjoys interactions with mother or primary caregiver

Motor
- Brings hands together, or to mouth
- Lifts head and pushes on arms when on tummy
- Reaches for objects
- Turns or makes crawling movement when on tummy

Language
- Turns head to follow familiar voices
- Laughs and squeals
- Combines sounds more often (for example, "aaah-oooh," "gaaa-gooo")

Activities
- Grasps more and reaches for objects
- Brings objects to mouth
- Increases activity when sees a toy

Social/Emotional
- Is increasingly interactive and comfortable with parents and caregivers
- Shows interest in mirrors, smiles and is playful
- Is able to comfort himself

At 4 months
(16 weeks)

At 6 months

Motor
- Puts weight on feet when held standing up
- Sits by himself
- Bangs and shakes objects
- Transfers objects from one hand to another
- Holds 2 objects at a time, one in each hand
- Rolls over from tummy to back

Language
- Responds to his name, turns and looks
- Babbles, making sounds like "da," "ga," "ba," "ka"

Activities
- Pays attention to what toys can do (for example, make music and light up)
- Looks toward object that drops out of sight

Social/Emotional
- Is becoming more aware of surroundings
- Notices if parents are present (or not)
- Reacts differently to strangers
- Expresses excitement, happiness, and unhappiness

Until age 2 years, adjust your child's age so his growth and progress takes into account that he was born early.

At 9 months

Motor
- Picks up small objects with thumb and finger
- Moves more easily (crawls, moves along furniture, walks when hand is held)
- Pulls to a stand

Language
- Recognizes familiar words (his name and phrases, such as "time for bath" and "go bye-bye")
- Babbles with combination of vowel and consonant sounds (for example, "dada," "baba," "mama")
- Imitates sounds and movements

Activities
- Explores objects carefully (turns them upside down, puts hands inside openings)
- Is more involved in feedings (tries to hold bottle or pick up finger foods)
- Resists toy being taken away

Social/Emotional
- Plays peek-a-boo and claps hands with excitement
- May show anxiety around strangers

Motor
- Stands alone
- Takes first steps
- Turns pages of a book a few at a time
- Puts small objects in container

Language
- Combines movements with sounds (reaches for an object and uses voice at same time)
- Pauses or stops when told not to do something
- Associates "mama" or "dada" with parents
- Uses one word again and again
- Hands you an object when asked

Activities
- Is better able to feed himself (tries to drink from cup)
- Helps with dressing

Social/Emotional
- Prefers to be with parents and caregivers
- Plays with other children

At 12 months
(1 year)

At 15 months
(1¼ years)

Motor
- Walks without help
- Climbs on chairs and other furniture

Language
- Uses 2 words besides "mama" and "dada"
- Asks for food or drink with sounds or words
- Shows what he wants by pulling, pointing, or grunting

Activities
- Feeds self with spoon, often insisting on feeding self

Social/Emotional
- Gives kisses
- Greets people with "hi"
- Listens to a story

Motor

- Scribbles
- Walks without help and can sometimes run
- Kicks ball forward
- Pulls a toy along the ground

At 18 months
(1½ years)

Language

- Follows simple directions, such as "give it to daddy"
- Says an increasing number of simple words (at least 5-10)
- Points to nose, mouth, eyes, ears, hands, and feet

Activities

- Enjoys eating by himself, but is messy
- Shows how objects work in "pretend" play (feeds a doll, pours tea into cup, brushes hair)

Social/Emotional

- Sometimes says no when interfered with
- Can separate from parent more easily, but happy when sees parent again

At 24-30 months
(2 to 2½ years)

Motor

- Scribbles in circular motion and can draw vertical lines
- Runs well, seldom falls
- Walks up and down stairs alone
- Stands on one foot without support
- Turns single pages in a book

Language

- Talks in 2- to 3-word sentences
- Follows 2-part instructions
- Uses at least 20 words (including pronouns he, she, I)

Activities

- Reads books by turning pages and looking at pictures
- Opens door by turning knob
- Washes and dries hands
- Feeds himself with little mess

Social/Emotional

- Helps with simple household tasks
- Usually responds to a correction by stopping

Motor
- Pedals tricycle
- Cuts with small scissors
- Draws or copies a complete circle
- Jumps in place, balances on one foot

Language
- Talks clearly (is understandable most of the time)
- Understands prepositions like "in," "on," "under," "beside"
- Combines sentences using and, or, but

Activities of Daily Living
- Is toilet trained and washes face and hands
- Gets dressed with help

Social/Emotional
- Gives direction to other children
- Plays a role in pretend games (mom, dad, teacher)

At 2 1/2 to 3 Years

At 3 1/2 Years

Motor
- Hops briefly on one foot
- Cuts paper with scissors

Language
- Identifies 4 colors correctly
- Knows concept of size, shape, number
- Counts 5 or more objects when asked, "How many?"

Activities
- Washes face without help
- Dresses and undresses without help, except for shoelaces

Social/Emotional
- Plays cooperatively with little conflict and supervision
- Pretend play is well developed

At 4 Years

Motor
- Hops on one foot repeatedly for a few seconds
- Skips or makes running broad jumps
- Draws recognizable pictures
- Draws a person with at least 3 parts (head, eyes, nose)

Language
- Follows a series of 3 simple instructions
- Reads a few letters
- Speaks in full sentences and is easily understood
- Makes conversation and tells stories of daily life

Activities
- Buttons one or more buttons
- Usually looks both ways before crossing street

Social/Emotional
- Is protective toward younger children
- Follows simple rules in board or card games

At 5 Years

Motor
- Swings on swing by himself
- Prints first name

Language
- Tells meaning of familiar words
- Recognizes most letters of the alphabet

Activities
- Goes to the toilet without any help

Social/Emotional
- Shows leadership among other children
- Plays dress up and make-believe

At School Age

Ongoing Issues Your Child May Face

As premature babies get older, some of them may face ongoing physical problems (for example, asthma or cerebral palsy). They also may face developmental challenges (for example, difficulties paying attention or lack of motor control). This may be especially true for babies who were very small at birth.

Once your child reaches school age, it will be important for you to work closely with his teacher and other school staff to identify any areas of concern. They also can help you find the right resources for help. If the school does not have the resources necessary for your child, his teachers can help you find local groups or programs to help him do well in school. You are not alone–your child's teachers and health care professionals are dedicated to helping you meet all his health and educational needs.

All babies will babble before they say real words. All babies will pull up to a stand before they walk. We are sure that babies will develop in these patterns. However, babies can reach these stages in different ways and at different times. This is especially true if they were born prematurely. Take some time to think about your baby's development and answer the questions below. Your answers will help he is going to grow.

- How does my baby like to communicate?
- How does he let me know what he is thinking and feeling?

- How does my baby like to explore how to use his body?
  Does he prefer using his fingers and hands (small muscles)?
  Does he prefer using his arms and legs (large muscles)?

- How does my baby respond to new situations? Does he jump right in? Does he prefer to hang back and look around before he feels safe?

- How does my baby like to explore? What kinds of objects and activities interest him? What do those interests tell me about him?

- What are my child's strengths? In what ways does he need more support?

Common Conditions, Concerns, and Equipment in the NICU

Babies in the NICU are carefully monitored because of their health risk. While the following is a comprehensive list of common conditions found in the NICU, it is by no means meant to scare parents. Not all preemies will have these problems, but, if your baby does have a common condition, the following explanation is meant to help you understand what is happening and calm your fears.

General Conditions

Prematurity

Babies born before 37 completed weeks of gestation (or before the 37th week of pregnancy) are called "preterm" or "premature." Preterm babies are at risk for a variety of problems, including the following:

- Breathing
- Feeding (and breathing and feeding at the same time)
- Infection
- Staying warm

Premature babies need special medical care that is offered only within Neonatal Intensive Care Units (NICUs) or Special Care Nurseries (SCNs).

Heart and blood pressure monitors

In the NICU, a baby's heart rate, respiratory (breathing) rate, blood pressure, and temperature all will be monitored. Small sticky pads are placed on the baby's skin and these detect information and send it to a screen at the baby's bedside. A small blood pressure cuff is used to measure blood pressure. This is also hooked up to the machine. Sometimes blood pressure is monitored through a thin tube inserted into an artery. An alarm will sound whenever the baby needs to be checked by a nurse but some alarms are "false alarms" caused by the baby's movements.

Central line

When your baby is born, the health care team may place a thin tube, called a central line or catheter, in the umbilical vein. This line is used to give your baby intravenous nutrition and medicine. The line also can be used to check how your baby is breathing. Later, your baby might need to have the umbilical line replaced with a PICC (peripherally inserted central catheter) line, which is placed in one of the major blood vessels. Other types of central lines, such as Hickman and Broviac catheters, also may be needed.

Hyperbilirubinemia (Jaundice)

Hyperbilirubinemia or jaundice occurs when there is too much of a chemical called bilirubin in the blood. Bilirubin is made when red blood cells (RBCs) are broken down after normal use, as is common after a baby is born, or from an infection or problem with the blood. High levels of bilirubin cause the skin to become yellow or pink-yellow in color. The more bilirubin, the more yellow (or jaundiced) the skin. If the bilirubin level becomes very, very high, it can cause more serious problems, like brain damage or hearing loss.

In a healthy baby, bilirubin moves through the blood to the liver and then leaves the body in the urine and stool. Because preemies have immature livers, there is a delay in how fast the bilirubin leaves the body. This can result in higher levels of bilirubin in a preemie than in a more mature baby. Bilirubin levels also can be higher in babies who are sick.

Bilirubin levels are measured in the blood shortly after birth and then every day until the levels begin to drop. Treatment for high bilirubin levels depends on the baby's weight and age. It usually includes using special blue lights, called phototherapy or "bili lights." These lights change the bilirubin to make it more soluble so it can easily leave the body in the urine. During this treatment, the baby will lie under the lights. His eyes will be protected and his position will be changed frequently to expose all skin areas. How high the bilirubin levels are determines
the number of lights a baby needs. If the phototherapy lights don't adequately decrease bilirubin levels, another treatment, called an exchange transfusion, can be done. This procedure is only rarely needed and involves exchanging some of the baby's blood with donated blood to lower the bilirubin level.

Infection (Sepsis)

Sepsis is an infection of the bloodstream. Usually, it is caused by germs (bacteria). In some cases, it is caused by a virus or fungus.

Sepsis can be very serious and often requires additional care or longer hospital stays. When babies get ill in the first week after birth, the infection might have started before birth or during delivery. Babies who become ill after 7 days of age have what is known as late-onset sepsis. This infection is usually caused from germs the baby is exposed to in the hospital. Premature babies are at risk for infection because of their fragile skin and poor ability to fight off germs. Possible signs of sepsis include the following:

- Body temperature that is too high or too low
- Breathing problems (such as apnea, or the need for oxygen or ventilator)
- Change in blood pressure (especially low blood pressure)
- Low activity level or decreased movement
- Feeding problems

Treatment for sepsis includes

- Antibiotics
- Blood tests to check for signs of infection
- Fluids or medicine to increase blood pressure
- Giving oxygen or using a ventilator to help the baby breathe

How long this treatment is needed depends on how sick the baby is and what caused the sepsis.

Temperature control

Healthy full-term babies have a layer of fat under the skin that protects them from heat loss. Babies who are born early have not had the chance to put on weight and do not have this fat layer under their skin. The best way to keep preterm babies warm is through the use of an isolette (or incubator). This is a special crib that provides extra heat to preemie or sick babies. As the baby gets bigger and more mature, he will be able to move into an open crib. This is one of the main criteria used to determine when a baby is ready to go home.

Radiant warmer

This is an open bed with a heat source over the baby. It may be used instead of an incubator, especially for babies who need frequent handling or care.

Late Onset Hearing Loss: Extended Stay in NICU

Left undetected, hearing loss in infants can negatively impact speech and language acquisition, academic achievement, and social and emotional development. If detected early, however, morbidity can be diminished and even eliminated through early intervention services. The following will review some of the risk factors associated with hearing loss that accompany an infant's extended stay in the NICU.

Very Low Birth Weight (<1,500 g)

The risk for sensorineural hearing loss increases as the birth weight decreases. Babies who weigh less than 3,000 g are also at an increased risk for hearing loss compared with babies weighing more than 3,000 g.

Ototoxic Drugs

Ototoxic drugs can cause toxic reactions to structures of the inner ear that can result in loss of hearing and/or balance. Following is an example of an ototoxic drug:

- Aminoglycoside antibiotics may be ototoxic when administered to a child, or to the fetus when administered to a pregnant woman. Sensorineural hearing loss results from damage to the hair cells of the vestibular and cochlear organs (components of the inner ear).

Low Apgar Score (0-4 at 1 minute or 1-6 at 5 minutes)

Newborns with low Apgar scores are at an increased risk for hearing loss because of their existing condition or because of consequential medical procedures.

Postnatal Infection Associated With Sensorineural Hearing Loss (Sepsis, Bacterial Meningitis)

Bacterial meningitis and sepsis are severe invasive disease. These infections can lead to sensorineural hearing loss. In addition, antibiotics used to treat the infections may be ototoxic.

Hyperbilirubinemia Requiring Exchange Transfusion

Hyperbilirubinemia, or jaundice, occurs in 50% to 60% of all newborns. It is often without consequence, but it can cause damage to the nervous system if severe. In cases of severe hyperbilirubinemia, the auditory neural pathways (cochlear nuclei of the brain stem) and/or the cochlea may be affected, leading to neonatal hearing loss. Babies with hyperbilirubinemia at a serum level requiring exchange transfusion should have additional auditory brainstem response (ABR) testing.

Mechanical Ventilation for >5 Days

By the time a baby has been put on mechanical ventilation, he may have already sustained a high level of oxygen deprivation. A lack of oxygen can accelerate the deterioration of the sensory cells of the inner ear. Mechanical ventilation also could indicate other possible problems associated with hearing loss, such as bronchiopulmonary dysplasia or persistent pulmonary hypertension.

Condition at Birth Requiring Use of Extracorporeal Membrane Oxygenation (ECMO)

Babies who need ECMO may experience levels of oxygen deprivation sufficient to cause damage to the sensory cells of the inner ear. About one-fourth of ECMO graduates develop sensorineural hearing loss. Roughly one-half of ECMO graduates with sensorineural hearing loss have a progressive type of loss, which reinforces the importance of follow-up screening.

(Permission to use information from *Risk Factors for Late Onset Hearing Loss: Extended Stay in NICU* was granted by Washington State Department of Health/Early Hearing Loss, Detection, Diagnosis, and Intervention Program.)

Breathing Conditions

Apnea and Bradycardia

It is normal for premature babies to have breathing pauses. Any pause in breathing that lasts for more than 20 seconds is called apnea. A decrease in the heart rate below a normal level is called bradycardia. These conditions are common in preemies and usually go away when they are between 35 and 40 weeks' corrected age. However, apnea might take longer to go away in infants born very preterm (23-27 weeks' gestation). These conditions are common in preemies because the part of the brain that controls breathing is not fully developed. They can cause the baby to become pale purple or dusky blue in color. The baby also might become limp and the heart rate might slow down.

Babies in the NICU are watched closely for apnea and bradycardia (often called A's and B's). When a baby stops breathing or the heart rate drops below a certain number, a monitor will alarm.

There are several types of treatment. First, if the apnea and bradycardia are mild, the baby simply may need to be observed or gently reminded to breathe by touching the baby or changing his position. If the baby is very premature or the apnea and bradycardia are severe, medicine (usually caffeine) is used. Otherwise, babies are treated with oxygen or air blowing in a little tube under the nose or with breathing support, such as CPAP or a ventilator.

Early Lung Conditions

Respiratory Distress Syndrome (RDS)

Another term that you may hear is respiratory distress syndrome (or RDS). It also might be called by its old name (hyaline membrane disease) or its biological cause (surfactant deficiency). RDS is very common in preemies. It affects babies whose lungs have lower than normal amounts of a body substance called surfactant. This substance helps make breathing easier by holding open the air sacs of the lungs. If these sacs do not open easily, the lungs cannot take in air, get oxygen into the bloodstream, or get rid of carbon dioxide. Babies with RDS breathe fast, causing the chest and ribs to pull in and out. They also may make grunting or soft crowing sounds when they breathe.

Tests to diagnose RDS include a chest x-ray and blood tests to measure oxygen and carbon dioxide levels (this test is called a "blood gas"). Any baby with trouble breathing should be checked for RDS.

Treatment includes giving the baby oxygen. This can be done with an oxygen hood or with CPAP (continuous positive airway pressure). CPAP is a scuba-like mask or nasal prongs that keep air sacs open and helps the baby breathe. If oxygen isn't enough, a ventilator (breathing machine) is needed. To breathe on a ventilator, a tube must be placed into the baby's airway (trachea). This tube is needed both to give surfactant and help with breathing. There are a number of different ventilators that may be used. Some give the baby regular breaths, others allow the baby to breathe on his own, and still others use gentle vibration to help the lungs. Up to 4 doses of surfactant can be given over the first 2 days after birth.

Complications of RDS can include lung collapse (or pneumothorax), intraventricular hemorrhage (IVH), developmental delay, and chronic lung disease (CLD), also called bronchopulmonary dysplasia (BPD).

Pneumothorax (Air Leaks or Lung Collapse)

A pneumothorax is an event that occurs when the breathing sacs in the lungs break and air leaks into and gets trapped in the space between the lung and the chest wall. If this happens, air cannot get back into the lungs for normal breathing. It can cause collapse of the lung as well. This condition is common in preemies or babies whose lungs lack surfactant. Babies who breathe in meconium (the first stool) while still in the womb are also at high risk for pneumothorax.

There are 3 types of air leaks that are seen in babies.

- "Spontaneous" pneumothorax, which occurs for no known reason in healthy babies and may or may not cause a problem.

- "Tension" pneumothorax, which is more common in babies who are on ventilators. This is a medical emergency because the lung collapse puts pressure on the heart, interfering with heart function and circulation.

- Pulmonary Interstitial Emphysema (PIE), which is a condition involving air leaking within the lung tissue itself. This type of air leak also puts the baby at increased risk of a pneumothorax and often requires the use of a special ventilator, especially the high frequency ventilator.

Tests include the use of fiber-optic lights (transillumination) to look for trapped air in the lungs and chest x-rays.

Treatment includes giving the baby high amounts of oxygen. A tension pneumothorax is treated with a chest tap (called a thoracentesis) to remove the air. If the air leak is severe, a chest tube is placed between the lung and chest wall to refill the lungs and allow them to heal over a few days.

Persistent Pulmonary Hypertension of the Newborn (Also Known as PPHN or Persistent Fetal Circulation)

Before birth, babies get oxygen from their mothers through the placenta. Therefore, they do not use their lungs to breathe air (although they make breathing movements, even when they are in the womb). When a baby is born, blood flows to the lungs and the baby breathes on his own. There are a number of conditions that can interrupt this process. These include

- Infection
- Meconium aspiration (when a baby breathes in a small amount of stool while still in the womb)
- Low oxygen levels
- Lack of surfactant in the lungs

If blood does not go to the lungs, the baby does not have enough oxygen. This causes the baby's skin color to be bluish-gray.

Tests include checking the baby's blood oxygen, pH, and carbon dioxide (blood gases), chest x-rays, and a special study of baby's heart called an echocardiogram (echo). This test checks the structure of the heart and lungs and blood pressure.

Treatments include using a ventilator to help the baby breathe, blood pressure medicine, a medicine that relaxes the lung blood pressure (called nitric oxide), and, in some cases, heart-lung bypass (extracorporeal membrane oxygenation).

Transient Tachypnea of the Newborn (TTN)

Tachypnea is the medical word for fast or rapid breathing. Rapid breathing that gets better over the first few hours or days and does not recur is called Transient Tachypnea of the Newborn (TTN). TTN occurs because fluid in the baby's lungs is not absorbed after birth. The symptoms of TTN are similar to RDS, but are usually are milder. Some babies with TTN need oxygen, but only rarely will a baby with TTN need to be on a ventilator.

Oxygen Hood and Nasal Cannula

An oxygen hood is a clear plastic box that goes over a baby's head. A nasal cannula is a thin tube with 2 small prongs that fit into a baby's nostrils. Both give oxygen to help with breathing.

Pulse Oximeter

To measure a baby's pulse, a small stretchy bandage with a sensor in it is wrapped around the baby's foot, hand, or wrist. The oximeter uses a light sensor to make sure there is enough oxygen in the baby's blood. The sensor does not hurt the baby and it helps the health care team know if the baby needs more or less oxygen.

Later Lung Conditions

Bronchopulmonary Dysplasia (BPD)

This also is known as chronic lung disease (CLD) of prematurity. BPD is most common in newborns who

- Lack surfactant in their lungs
- Have very underdeveloped lungs
- Need high amounts of oxygen
- Are on a ventilator

The highest rates of BPD are among newborns born at 23 to 26 weeks of gestation (14-17 weeks before their due date). However, it can occur in other preterm newborns as well. Rarely, BPD can affect ill full-term newborns.

Treatment includes giving the baby oxygen, good nutrition, and sometimes diuretics (medicine that increases urine output) or bronchodilators (medicine that helps open the airways). A baby with BPD might need to be on a ventilator for a while before he can breathe on his own. After the ventilator is removed, the baby still will need to get oxygen through a little tube under the nose. Some babies need to go home with this extra oxygen.

A baby with BPD must be protected from catching a cold or the flu. For these babies, a simple cold can turn into a severe, or even fatal, pneumonia. While many babies with BPD outgrow their lung problems, some preemies with BPD will have lung problems that last through young adulthood.

Pneumonia: This lung infection is common in premature and other sick babies. A baby's doctors may suspect pneumonia if the baby has difficulty breathing, if his rate of breathing changes, or if he has an increased number of apnea episodes.

The doctor will listen to the baby's lungs with a stethoscope and then do an X-ray to see if there is excess fluid in the lungs. Sometimes, the doctor may insert a thin tube down the windpipe (trachea) to take a sample of the lung fluid. The fluid is then tested to see what type of bacterium or virus is causing the infection, so that the doctor can choose the most effective drug to treat it. Babies with pneumonia generally are treated with antibiotics. They also may need additional oxygen until the infection clears up.

Heart Conditions

Patent Ductus Arteriousus (PDA)

Before birth, babies get oxygen from their mothers. They do not use their lungs to breathe. Instead, blood goes past the lungs through an opening in a blood vessel just outside the heart called the ductus arteriosus. During the first few hours or days after birth, this opening starts to close, allowing the baby to use the lungs to breathe. However, it is not uncommon for the ductus arteriousus to stay open in sick or premature babies. If that happens, it is called a patent ductus arteriosus or PDA. (The ductus is actually a normal fetal artery connecting the aorta and the pulmonary artery.)

In a PDA, extra fluid builds up in the lungs, making it hard for the baby to breathe. Symptoms include

- Fast breathing
- Need of a ventilator (breathing machine)
- Poor growth
- Presence of a heart murmur

Treatment depends on how the baby is affected by the PDA. A cardiologist (heart doctor) will examine the baby and use a heart test called an echocardiogram to confirm the PDA. A medicine may be used to close the PDA. In some cases, the baby might need to have surgery to close the PDA.

Congenital Heart Defects

Congenital Heart Defects are structural heart problems that are present at birth. They originate in the first weeks of pregnancy when the heart is forming.

Coarctation of the aorta: The aorta is the large artery that sends blood from the heart to the rest of the body. In this condition, the aorta may be too narrow for the blood to flow evenly. A surgeon can remove the narrow part and connect the ends together, replace the constricted section with man-made material, or patch it with part of a blood vessel taken from elsewhere in the
body. Sometimes, this narrowed area can be widened by inflating a balloon on the tip of a catheter inserted through an artery.

Heart valve abnormalities: Some babies are born with heart valves that are narrowed, closed, or blocked, and prevent blood from flowing smoothly. Some babies may require placement of a shunt (tube between 2 blood vessels) to allow blood to bypass the blockage until the baby is big enough to have the valve repaired or replaced.

Septal defects: A septal defect refers to a hole in the wall (septum) that divides the 2 upper or lower chambers of the heart. Because of this hole, the blood cannot circulate as it should, and the heart has to work extra hard. A surgeon can close the hole by sewing or patching it. Small holes might close by themselves and not need repair at all.

Tetralogy of Fallot: In this condition, a combination of 4 structural problems keeps the normal amount of blood from getting to the lungs. As a result, the baby has episodes of cyanosis (blue spells) and may grow poorly. New surgical techniques allow early repair of this complex heart defect.

Transposition of the great arteries: Here, the positions of the 2 major arteries leaving the heart are reversed. Each artery arises from the wrong pumping chamber. Surgical advances have enabled correction of this problem in the newborn period.

Intestinal Conditions

Necrotizing Enterocolitis (NEC)

NEC is a serious disease of the intestines that most often affects premature babies; however, sometimes full-term babies also get NEC. Babies who are born very early, are very small, or are very sick are at highest risk. This is because they often have less blood flow to their intestines and are at higher risk for infection.

NEC usually develops within the first 3 weeks, often after feedings are started. The intestine becomes smaller and weaker, and this can cause a hole to form. If a hole (perforation) develops, bacteria can leak into the baby's blood or abdomen, causing a life-threatening infection.

NEC can happen very quickly–within a few hours. The baby can go from healthy to critically ill. When a baby recovers from NEC, the bowel may still be weak and additional problems can come up when feedings are started again. However, it is rare for NEC to happen again.

Tests include abdominal x-rays and blood tests.

Treatment includes giving the baby IV fluids and antibiotics. Babies with NEC have a tube inserted to drain stomach acid and are fed through an IV to let the bowels rest (often for 1 to 2 weeks). Surgery is needed if the disease is severe or a perforation (hole) is found in the intestine.

Blood Conditions

Anemia

Anemia is the term for a low blood count or low red blood cells. Red blood cells are important because they carry oxygen throughout the body. Preemies are at higher risk for anemia because of their size and because of the number of blood tests they need. If anemia is severe or the baby also has low blood pressure, a blood transfusion is needed. Less severe anemia is treated by giving iron medicine and by adding iron to breast milk or formula.

Neurological Conditions

Intraventricular Hemorrhage (IVH)

An IVH is a collection of blood (hemorrhage) in or around the normally fluid-filled spaces (ventricles) on each side of the brain. It is common in very small and very sick preemies because the blood vessels on their brains are very delicate and can break easily. Babies with breathing problems and low blood pressure are at especially high risk for IVH. Most hemorrhages occur in the first few days of life. Babies born before 32 weeks' gestation have a special test of the head (called a sonogram or ultrasound) by the seventh day of age. IVH is divided into the following grades (or degrees):

Grade 1: A small amount of blood outside the ventricles

Grade 2: Bleeding inside the ventricles but the ventricles are normal size

Grade 3: Blood inside the ventricles and the ventricles are large in size

Grade 4: Bleeding outside the ventricles into the surrounding brain tissue

Major bleeding can cause increased pressure on the brain. It also can cause not enough blood to go to the brain tissue. Brain bleeding in premature babies can have a variety of long-term effects. Some babies will not have any permanent damage and will develop normally. Other babies can have mild, moderate, or severe brain damage.

Brain and Body Imaging

There are several types of tests that your baby may need to help doctors see inside the body, including the following:

- Ultrasound: Takes pictures of the internal organs using sound waves. It does not hurt and can be done at the baby's bedside.

- X-rays: Takes pictures of the lungs, bones, and other internal organs. Several x-rays might be needed depending on what the doctor is looking for. The baby will be exposed to a small amount of radiation during an x-ray. However, x-rays are often needed to help make important decisions about a baby's care. They also can be done at the bedside.

- Computed tomography (CT or CAT scan): Takes more detailed pictures than an x-ray or ultrasound. A beam of energy is focused on a certain area of the body and then shown in detail on a computer. This test cannot be done at the baby's bedside and involves greater radiation exposure than a regular x-ray.

- Magnetic resonance imaging (MRI): Uses powerful magnets and computers to create images of tissue that are even more detailed then a CT scan. This test cannot be done at the baby's bedside. Some babies need sedation to help keep them still during this test. An MRI does not give the baby any radiation exposure.

Periventricular Leukomalacia (PVL)

PVL is a cyst formation in the brain tissue around the ventricles (chambers) in the brain. PVL may be caused by

- A hemorrhage in the brain

- A brain infection, such as meningitis

- Other infections, including infections during prenatal life

It can occur in premature babies and usually happens without warning. It can be seen with a head ultrasound, although it may take several weeks before PVL shows up. PVL increases the risk of a baby having long-term problems with muscle movement and coordination, vision, or intellectual development.

Retinopathy of Prematurity (ROP)

This is an abnormal growth of blood vessels in the retina (the lining at the back of the eyeball that sends images to the brain). It is seen in some preterm babies, especially those born more than 12 weeks early.

When a baby is born early, the blood vessels in the eyes are not fully developed. If these blood vessels do not grow normally, bleeding and scarring can affect vision. Doctors do not know all the reasons why ROP happens, but being premature and the use of high amounts of oxygen are 2 risk factors. This is why oxygen levels for preemies are tightly controlled.

ROP is more common in very small and very premature babies. If your baby was born before 30 weeks' gestation, he will need to see a specially trained eye doctor called an ophthalmologist. The doctor will look at the development of your baby's retina (eye). Regular eye examinations will be needed until the retina is fully developed. Severe ROP can lead to vision problems and even blindness. Treatment may involve laser surgery or cryosurgery to stop the blood vessels from growing abnormally.

Preemie Care
Glossary of
NICU Terms

*Glossary definitions adapted
from the March of Dimes and
Mothers of Super Twins (MOST)*

A

ABO incompatibility:
Blood incompatibility between the mother and fetus that can result in destruction of fetal red blood cells, jaundice, and anemia.

Adjusted Age:
Used most appropriately to describe children up to 3 years of age who were born preterm. "Corrected age" or "adjusted age" is calculated by subtracting the number of weeks born before 40 weeks of gestation from the chronological age.

Anemia:
One of the more common blood disorders, anemia occurs when the level of healthy red blood cells (RBCs) in the body becomes too low.

Apgar Score:
A scoring system that helps the physician estimate a baby's general condition at birth. The test measures a baby's heart rate, breathing, muscle tone, reflex response, and color at 1 minute, 5 minutes, and 10 minutes of life. Named after its creator, Virginia Apgar.

Apnea:
A pause in breathing that lasts longer than 20 seconds. Apnea of Prematurity occurs in babies who are born prematurely (before 34 weeks of gestation). Because the brain or respiratory system may be immature or underdeveloped, the baby may not be able to regulate his or her own breathing. (Apnea monitor: Machine that detects interruptions in breathing.)

Artery:
Blood vessel that carries oxygen to all parts of the body.

Asphyxia:
Lack of oxygen.

Aspiration:
Inhaling a foreign object, such as food, medicine, or meconium.

Attending Physician:
The physician who has been selected by or assigned to the patient and who has assumed primary responsibility for the treatment and care of the patient.

Audiologist:
A medical professional with 6 years of training who treats patients with hearing, balance, and related ear problems.

Bagging:
Pumping air or oxygen into a baby's lungs by squeezing a bag or air into a mask placed over the baby's mouth and nose, or through an endotracheal tube.

Betamethasone:
Corticosteroid given to the mother before the baby is born to stimulate fetal lung maturation and to decrease the frequency and damage from intracranial hemorrhage in premature babies.

Bilirubin:
Bilirubin is a breakdown product of hemoglobin, the substance in blood that carries oxygen. Normally, bilirubin passes through the liver and is excreted as bile through the intestine. Jaundice occurs when bilirubin builds up faster than a newborn's liver can break it down and pass it from the body. (Bililights: Blue fluorescent lights used to treat jaundice.)

Birth Defect:
Abnormality of structure, function, or body metabolism (inborn error of body chemistry) present at birth that results in physical and/or mental disability, or is fatal.

Blood Gases:
Levels of oxygen and carbon dioxide in the blood.

Bradycardia:
A heart rate of less than 100 beats per minute, slower than normal for a baby.

Breast Pump:
A machine to collect breast milk without the baby present. A hospital-grade breast pump is often more powerful than those for home use, and may be available for rental.

Bronchopulmonary Dysplasia (BPD):
A chronic lung disorder that is most common among children who were born prematurely, with low birth weights, and who received prolonged mechanical ventilation.

Cannula:
A slender tube that sits below the nose and can be used to deliver oxygen.

Cardiopulmonary Monitor:
Machine that tracks heart and breathing rates.

Catheter:
A hollow, flexible tube for insertion into a body cavity, duct, or vessel to allow the passage of fluids, or distend or drain a passageway or body cavity. Its uses include delivery of intravenous fluids, the drainage of urine from the bladder through the urethra or insertion through a blood vessel into the heart for diagnostic purposes.

Central Venous Line:
A narrow tube that is placed into a blood vessel and passed into a larger blood vessel in the chest or abdomen. It is used to receive medicine, IV nutrition, and to draw blood.

Cerebral Palsy (CP):
Appearing in the first few years of life, this diagnosis means the child will have abnormal muscle tone (too tight or too loose) and might also have problems moving parts of their body. The extent of the problem may not be fully known until about age 2 years.

Chicken Pox (Varicella):
Common childhood illness characterized by an itchy rash and fever. When contracted by a pregnant woman, it can occasionally cause birth defects or severe newborn illness. Chicken pox is highly contagious.

CPAP (Continuous Positive Airway Pressure):
Air is delivered to a baby's lungs either through small tubes in the baby's nose or through a tube that has been inserted into his windpipe. The tubes are attached to a ventilator, which helps the baby breathe, but does not breathe for him.

Complete Blood Count (CBC):
Blood test that looks at the number and type of white blood cells (infection-fighting cells), the concentration of hemoglobin, the percentage of blood volume consisting of red blood cells (hematocrit, oxygen-carrying cells), and the number of platelets (blood-clotting cells).

Computed Tomography (CT or CAT Scan):
Imaging technique that produces precise pictures of tissue using a narrow beam of radiation and computer processing of a series of images.

Congenital Diaphragmatic Hernia:
Birth defect involving an opening in the diaphragm, the large muscle that separates the chest and abdomen. Abdominal organs, such as the stomach, liver, and intestines, can move through the opening into the chest, where they interfere with lung development.

Continuous Positive Airway Pressure (CPAP):
This machine pushes a continuous flow of air or oxygen, through small tubes that fit into the baby's nostrils (called nasal CPAP), to the airways to help keep tiny air passages in the lungs open.

Cryotherapy:
Freezing of abnormal tissue to halt its growth. This form of treatment can be used in severe cases of retinopathy of prematurity (ROP) but, more recently, cryotherapy for ROP has been largely replaced by laser therapy.

Cubic Centimeter (cc):
A metric unit of volume equal to one-thousandth of a liter (a milliliter). There are 30 cc in a fluid ounce.

Culture:
A laboratory test that detects infections in the body by placing samples in special nutrients that allow bacteria to grow. Most current culture systems monitor bacterial growth for up to 7 days.

Cyanosis:
A blue or gray discoloration of the skin caused by insufficient oxygen.

Cytomegalovirus (CMV):
A viral infection that, when contracted by a pregnant woman, can result in severe newborn illness, and sometimes lead to chronic disabilities such as mental retardation, or vision and hearing loss. CMV also can be acquired after birth and can lead to hearing loss.

D

Developmental Delays:
The failure to meet certain milestones, such as rolling, sitting, walking, and talking at the average age.

Developmental Pediatrician:
These physicians have 10 years of training and specialize in evaluating and treating problems with child development. They assess the level of development of premature babies from both the motor (movement) and intellectual (learning) viewpoints.

E

Early Intervention Program (EI):
Early intervention refers to services that are provided to children aged 3 years or younger, who have or might develop a special need that may affect their development.

Echocardiogram:
The use of ultrasound to view the structure and function of the heart.

Electrocardiogram (EKG):
Measurement of electrical activity of the heart from a number of specific viewpoints. This activity is detected through adhesive patches placed on the chest, arms, and legs.

Electrodes:
A conductor used to make contact with a nonmetallic part of a circuit.

Electroencephalogram (EEG):
A noninvasive and painless study, in which electrodes placed on the scalp record the electrical activity of the brain. To conduct their study, metal electrodes have to be temporarily glued to the scalp.

Endotracheal Tube (ET Tube):
A tube that is placed down a newborn's trachea (windpipe) and delivers warm humidified air and oxygen to the lungs.

Exchange Transfusion:
Special type of blood transfusion in which some of the baby's blood is removed and replaced with blood from a donor. It can be used to treat severe jaundice.

Extracorporeal Membrane Oxygenation (ECMO):
In babies, this machine usually is used to allow the lungs to rest and recover from disease or medical conditions. ECMO is similar to the heart-lung bypass that is used in the operating room for heart surgery, but, in newborns, it is used for longer periods of time. It is also called extracorporeal life support (ECLS).

Extremely Low Birth Weight:
Extremely low birth weight babies refer to babies with a birth weight of less than 1,000 g or 2 lbs 3 oz.

Extremely Premature:
Babies born between 23 and 27 weeks' gestation.

F

Failure to Thrive:
The failure to gain weight as expected, which is often accompanied by poor height growth.

Fellow:
Physician who has completed medical school, internship, and a residency, and currently is undergoing very specialized (subspecialty) training in one particular field of study. Neonatology fellows are training to become specialists in newborn medicine.

Fontanelle or Fontanel:
"Soft spot" between the parts of the baby's skull that will later grow together.

G

Gastroenterologist:
A physician with specialized training in diagnosing and treating diseases of the gastrointestinal (GI) tract and digestive system.

Gastroesophageal Reflux:
This occurs when gastric juice from the stomach backs up into the esophagus. Adults refer to this as "heartburn" although it has nothing to do with the heart.

Gastrointestinal Tract (GI Tract):
The tube that goes from the mouth to the anus where food is digested and eliminated from the body (as a bowel movement).

Gastroschisis:
Birth defect involving an opening in the abdominal wall, through which the abdominal organs bulge out, usually right beside the umbilical cord.

Gastrostomy:
Surgically created opening through the abdominal skin and into the stomach, through which a baby can be fed.

Gavage Feeding:
A method of feeding a baby with breast milk or formula before he has learned how to coordinate breathing and swallowing. A small flexible tube is placed into a baby's nostril or mouth and passed down into the stomach.

Gestation:
Period of time between last menstrual period and birth. In humans, 40 weeks is the average gestation for a full-term singleton. Commonly called pregnancy.

Gram:
A metric unit of weight equal to one thousandth of a kilogram. One gram weighs the same as one plain M&M's candy or one small paper clip. There are 30 grams in an ounce.

Group B Streptococcus:
Bacterial infection that a baby can contract as he passes through the birth canal, sometimes resulting in further illness. Many cases can be prevented by screening and/or treating infected women with antibiotics during labor and delivery.

H

Heart Failure:
When the heart cannot pump enough blood to meet the body's needs.

Hematocrit:
The percentage of blood volume consisting of red blood cells. Used as a measure of anemia.

Hemoglobin:
The component of red blood cells that carries oxygen. Used as a measure of anemia.

Herpes Simplex:
Virus that can be transmitted sexually, sometimes causing genital sores in infected adults. The virus can occupy the mouth, the genitals, or birth canal; on the lips it causes "cold sores." A baby may become infected passing through an infected birth canal, sometimes resulting in severe newborn illness or future medical problems.

Hernia:
The protrusion of an organ or structure through muscles that usually contain them.

High-Frequency Ventilation:
Special form of mechanical ventilation, designed to help reduce complications to the infant's delicate lungs. It provides rapid respiratory rates. Often called an Oscillator or Jet Ventilator (respirator).

Hydrocephalus:
A condition where too much fluid collects in the ventricles, exerting increased pressure on the brain and causing the baby's head to expand abnormally. Surgery may be required.

Hyperglycemia:
High blood glucose levels.

Hypoglycemia:
Low blood glucose levels.

I

Ileal Perforation:
A hole in part of the small intestine called the ileum.

Incubator/Isolette:
A heat-controlled crib used to maintain a baby's body temperature in the normal range.

Inflammation:
Pain, redness, and swelling, possibly caused by infection or injury.

Infusion Pump:
Device that delivers measured amounts of fluids or medications into the bloodstream over a period of time.

Intrauterine Growth Restriction (IUGR):
Inadequate growth of the fetus so that it is smaller than expected for gestational age. This can happen at any time during pregnancy.

Intravenous (IV):
A small tube inserted into a vein in the hand, foot, arm, leg, or scalp. An IV delivers medicine and/or fluids into the blood.

Intraventricular Hemorrhage (IVH):
Condition in which immature and fragile blood vessels within the brain bleed into the hollow chambers (ventricles) normally reserved for cerebrospinal fluid. Sometimes this bleeding also spreads into the tissue surrounding the ventricles. An IVH is assigned a grade to give an estimate of how serious it is.

Interval Delivery:
In multiple gestation, the delivery of a subsequent baby that is delayed after the preterm delivery of the first.

Intubation:
The procedure of inserting a tube through the mouth or nose, down the throat, and into the trachea or windpipe of a patient who may have difficulty breathing or might be at risk of stopping breathing because of illness, surgery, or other medical problem.

Jaundice:
Yellow discoloration of skin and, sometimes, whites of the eyes that results from excess of a body chemical called bilirubin in the body's system. If it is significant, jaundice might require use of special lights (phototherapy) until the baby is more mature. Severe jaundice is treated with exchange transfusion. Also known as hyperbilirubinemia.

Kangaroo Care:
Holding a baby against one's naked chest, so there is skin-to-skin contact.

Lactation Consultant:
A health care professional (sometimes, but not always, a nurse) who provides information and support about breastfeeding and pumping breast milk.

Lanugo:
Fine, downy hair that covers the fetus until shortly before or after birth.

Lead Wires:
The wires that go from a monitor to its electrodes (sticky patches on the chest).

Lesion:
A patch of abnormal skin, or the part of an injury or infection that is abnormal and causes an illness.

Licensed Practical Nurse/Licensed Vocational Nurse:
Health care professional with a vocational education lasting approximately 12 months and licensed to give nursing care under the direct supervision of a registered nurse or physician. In some states, called a licensed vocational nurse.

Ligation:
The act of binding or of applying a tie, wire, or bandage around a limb or blood vessel to restrict blood flow. It is used to treat patent ductus anteriousus (PDA) among other uses.

Liquid Ventilation:
A form of respiration in which a machine is used to deliver an oxygen rich liquid, rather than air.

Low Birth Weight:
Low birth weight babies are born weighing less than 2,500 g or 5 lbs 8 oz at birth.

Lumbar Puncture:
A diagnostic procedure that is done to collect a sample of spinal fluid for analysis, or, on rare occasions, to relieve increased pressure in the spinal fluid. It is also known as a spinal tap.

M

Magnetic Resonance Imaging (MRI):
Imaging technique that uses powerful magnets and computers to produce a detailed picture of internal tissues and organs.

Mechanical Ventilation:
Using a ventilator to help a very sick baby breathe while his lungs recover.

Meconium:
Fecal material made by the fetus; usually passed in the first bowel movement after birth. Sometimes meconium is passed in the amniotic fluid before birth and inhaled in the amniotic fluid during the fetus's normal breathing movement.

Meconium Aspiration Syndrome (MAS):
Problems caused by meconium (baby's first bowel movement) going into the lungs while the baby is still in the womb. This can be serious but, usually, the baby eventually recovers fully.

Medicaid:
A program partially sponsored by the federal government and administered by states that is intended to provide health care and health-related services to both low-income individuals and other qualifying persons. A child may qualify regardless of parental income, based on medical circumstances, even if the child has other health insurance.

Meningitis:
An inflammation of the lining of the brain, usually from viral or bacterial infection.

Microcephaly:
A condition in which the circumference of the head is small because of abnormal brain growth. This condition might result in future cerebral palsy or learning problems.

Micropreemie:
A newborn who weighs less than 800 g or 1 lb 12 oz at birth.

Milestones:
Skills most children can perform at certain ages. Examples include smiling, rolling, sitting, scooting, crawling, standing, walking, and talking.

Monitor:
A machine that records information such as heartbeat, body temperature, respiration rate, and blood pressure.

Moro Reflex:
A normal reflex of young babies; a sudden loud noise causes the child to stretch out the arms and flex (scrunch up) the legs.

Myopia:
The inability to see distant objects as clearly as near objects.

N

Nasal Cannula:
The "oxygen tubes" that give extra oxygen by blowing moisturized oxygen, possibly mixed with air, into the nose.

Nasal Prongs:
Small plastic tubes that fit into or under a baby's nose to deliver oxygen.

Nasogastric Tube (NG Tube):
A tube that is passed through the nose and down through the throat and esophagus and into the stomach.

Nebulizer Treatment:
A device for giving medicine by making a fine mist that is inhaled through the nose and/or mouth.

Necrotizing Entercolitis (NEC):
An infection that destroys part of the baby's intestines. Drugs and/or surgery may be required.

Neonatal Intensive Care Unit (NICU):
There are 3 levels of NICUs. Level 3 NICUs care for any baby that may have, or could have, severe or life-threatening conditions. Level 2 NICUs care for any newborns that require monitoring after birth and more than routine newborn care. Level 1 NICUs deliver routine newborn care. Level 1 NICUs are usually reserved for full-term babies, and might not have specialized equipment or physicians specializing in newborn problems.

Neonatal Nurse Practitioner (NNP):
An advanced practice nurse with specialized training and expertise in neonatal care, NNPs are licensed to assess, diagnose, manage, and treat critically ill and convalescing neonates. In addition, NNPs prescribe medicine, write orders, interpret results, perform emergency and daily procedures, and attend high-risk deliveries.

Neonatologist:
Physician with 10 years of training specialized in dealing with the diseases and care of newborns.

Neurologist:
Physician with at least 3 years of post-medical school training specialized in dealing with the diseases and care of the brain and nerves.

NG Tube:
(see Nasogastric Tube)

Nitric Oxide:
A gas naturally produced by the body that can also be given as a medication that is breathed in and helps expand blood vessels. It is sometimes used to treat babies with persistent pulmonary hypertension of the newborn.

Noninvasive:
Something that does not enter the body through the skin or an opening (mouth, nose, anus, etc).

O

Occupational Therapist:
A health care professional with 4 to 6 years of training who helps people who are ill or disabled learn to manage their daily activities. In the NICU, OTs may be involved in giving the premature baby stimulation, helping the baby learn to coordinate sucking, breathing, and swallowing while helping the baby stay comfortable and relaxed. They also teach the parents about techniques to enhance infant development and other activities.

Ophthalmologist:
Physician (MD) specializing in diagnosis and treatment of eye diseases and disorders: refractive, medical, and surgical problems.

Orogastric Tube:
A flexible tube inserted through the mouth, down the throat and esophagus, and into the stomach.

Otoacoustic Emission Test (OAE):
A passive audiologic test that verifies cochlear activity; often used in testing babies suspected of hearing loss.

Oximeter (Pulse Oximeter):
A device worn on the finger, toe, or earlobe that painlessly measures levels of oxygen in the blood.

Oxygen Therapy:
Giving extra oxygen to the tissues of the body through the lungs in a number of ways, including through a ventilator (respirator), mask, nasal cannula, or plastic oxygen hood or tent. The amount of oxygen given may be measured as a percentage, and in number of liters, or milliliters, of flow per minute.

P

Patent Ductus Arteriosus (PDA):
A heart condition caused by the failure of a small blood vessel (the ductus arteriosus) to close. Usually, this normal opening between the aorta and the pulmonary artery closes just after birth. When it does not, the baby may be treated with medicine or surgery to fix the condition, to prevent too much blood from "flooding" the lungs.

Pediatrician:
Physician with at least 3 post-medical school years of training in the care and treatment of children.

Percutaneous Line/Percutaneous Central Catheter (PICC):
A long catheter placed into a surface vein, with the catheter tip extending farther into the body into a large central vein. A PICC does not have to be replaced as often as a regular IV line.

Periventricular Leukomalacia:
Changes, usually small cysts in brain tissue around the ventricles or fluid spaces of the brain. This cystic change is linked with an increased risk of future problems with learning, vision, or movement.

Persistent Pulmonary Hypertension of the Newborn (PPHN):

In PPHN, it is difficult for blood to get into the lungs and pick up more oxygen that can go to the rest of the body. The cause usually is unknown, and treatments are based on the individual situation. Persistent pulmonary hypertension (PPHN) is also known as Persistent Fetal Circulation (PFC).

Phototherapy:

Treatment for jaundice in a newborn. The newborn is placed under (or on top of) special lights to help the body break down the extra bilirubin in the blood.

Physical Therapist (PT):

A health care professional with 4 years or more of training who performs and teaches exercises and other physical activities to aid in rehabilitation and maximize physical muscle and movement development.

Physician:

A graduate of a medical school or school of osteopathy with an MD or DO degree.

Pneumothorax:

Air that has leaked from the baby's lungs and gets trapped in the space between the baby's lungs and chest wall. While small leaks usually cause no problems and require no treatment, larger leaks may cause serious complications, such as lung collapse, and require withdrawal of the air with a needle and syringe or a surgical procedure to place a tube to drain the trapped air and reinflate the lung.

Pulse Oximeter:

A small device that uses a light sensor to help determine blood oxygen levels.

R

Radiant Warmer:

A heater that works by sending out radiant energy, usually in the form of heat. It warms objects without needing to touch them. Radiant warmers are often used to maintain temperature of babies in the neonatal intensive care units.

Radiologist:

A physician with 7 seven years of training who specializes in creating and interpreting pictures of areas inside the body.

Registered Nurse:
Health care professional with 2 or 4 years of training who is licensed to treat patient responses to illness and to carry out medication regimens prescribed by a physician, nurse practitioner, dentist, or physician's assistant; usually has an associate's or bachelor's degree and may have additional degrees or certificates when working in the NICU.

Resident:
A physician with 4 years of training in medical or osteopathy school who is in the process of completing the additional 3 years of training in a primary specialty (for example, pediatrics, ophthalmology, radiology, obstetrics/gynecology) following medical school.

Respirator:
A machine that helps breathing by supplying and regulating a flow of air and oxygen that goes through a tube threaded through the nose or mouth, down the back of the throat, and into the trachea (windpipe). It is also called a ventilator.

Respiratory Distress Syndrome (RDS):
Condition in which a premature baby with immature lungs does not have sufficient surfactant, a protective film that helps air sacs in the lungs to stay open.

Respiratory Syncytial Virus (RSV):
A virus that causes a mild, cold-like illness in adults. In premature babies or full-term babies with lung problems, it can cause serious illness, such as bronchiolitis or pneumonia.

Respiratory Therapists:
A health care professional with 3 to 5 years of training who assesses breathing and heart function, treats with oxygen therapy or ventilation, and gives medicines to help with breathing as prescribed by a physician or practitioner.

Retina:
Lining at the rear of the eye that relays messages about what the eyes see to the brain.

Retinopathy of Prematurity (ROP):
A condition in which the blood vessels in the baby's eyes do not develop normally. This can reverse and normalize or progress to serious disease that can lead to hemorrhage, scarring, and/or retinal detachment that limit vision. ROP is treated with laser therapy.

Rh Disease:
Blood incompatibility between the mother and fetus that causes destruction of fetal red blood cells.

S

Sepsis:
A blood infection.

Small for Gestational Age (SGA):
Newborns whose birth weight is <10th percentile for their gestational age. If weight gain of the fetus is abnormal, this is called Intrauterine Growth Restriction (IUGR).

Social Worker:
A professional with 4 to 6 years of training who helps families cope with stress, crisis, and change. In the NICU setting, the social worker helps families access community resources such as support groups and assistance programs. Social workers help with planning the baby's hospital discharge.

Spina Bifida:
A birth defect involving the spinal cord, often resulting in varying degrees of paralysis, bladder, and bowel problems. Affected babies may require surgery during the newborn period to close the back and prevent further nerve damage and infection. Surgery cannot reverse nerve damage that already has occurred.

Step-down Unit:
Nursing unit with patients who are not in need of intensive care but still require skilled nursing care.

Supplemental Security Income (SSI):
A federal income program funded by general tax revenues. Parents of children who qualify, based on medical and financial criteria, receive monthly payments to assist with health care expenses.

Surfactant/Pulmonary Surfactant:
A protective substance that keeps small air sacs in the lungs from collapsing.

Syndrome:
A combination of signs and symptoms that, when present together, are associated with a specific medical condition.

Swaddling:
Wrapping babies snugly in cloths or blankets so that movement of the limbs is restricted, providing the baby with a secure womb-like feeling.

T

Tachycardia:
Rapid heart rate.

Tachypnea:
Rapid breathing.

Tonic Neck Reflex:
One of the reflexes present at birth, also called the fencing reflex. A newborn will bend one arm while the other is extended away from the body, in the direction the baby is facing.

Total Parenteral Nutrition (TPN):
A technique in which nutrients are given to a person through an intravenous infusion. TPN often requires a PICC or CVL.

Toxoplasmosis:
A parasitic infection that, when contracted by a pregnant woman, can result in serious newborn illness and chronic disabilities, such as intellectual disability, cerebral palsy, seizures, or vision and hearing loss.

Transfusion:
The transfer of whole blood or blood products from one individual to another.

Twin-Twin Transfusion Syndrome (TTTS):
A disease of the placenta (or afterbirth) that affects identical twin pregnancies. The shared placenta contains abnormal blood vessels that can convey blood from one twin to another, resulting in a higher red blood cell count and, sometimes, better growth, in one twin than another.

U

Ultrasound (Sonogram):
The use of ultrasonic waves for diagnostic or therapeutic purposes. In the NICU, ultrasound is used to obtain an image of an internal body structure.

Umbilical Arterial Catheter (UAC):
A line placed directly into the umbilical artery through the baby's umbilical cord.

Umbilical Venous Catheter (UVC):
A line placed directly into the umbilical vein (a much larger vein than a peripheral vein) through the baby's umbilical cord.

V

Vein:
A blood vessel leading toward the heart.

Ventilator:
Mechanical breathing machine.

Ventricle:
A small chamber, one of the central chambers in the brain, or one of the 2 lower chambers of the heart.

Very Low Birth Weight:
Very low birth weight babies weigh less than 1500 g or 3 lbs 5 oz.

Very Premature:
Babies born between 28 and 32 weeks' gestation.

Viable:
Viable means a newborn is potentially able to survive.

Vital Signs:
Temperature, heart rate, respiratory rate, and blood pressure.

W

Women, Infants, and Children Program (WIC):
WIC is a nutrition program that helps pregnant women, new mothers, and young children eat well and stay healthy. It provides food or formula to parents of babies.

Important Web Site Resources for Families

American Academy of Pediatrics (www.healthychildren.org)

AAP Section on Perinatal Pediatrics (www.aap.org/perinatal)

March of Dimes Parents (www.marchofdimes.com/pnhec/pnhec.asp)

National Association of Neonatal Nurses (www.nann.org)

Back to Sleep (www.healthychildcare.org/sids.html)

Bright Futures (http://brightfutures.aap.org)

Caring Bridge (www.caringbridge.org)

Cystic Fibrosis Foundation (www.cff.org/AboutCF)

Vaccine Info (www.cdc.gov/vaccines)

March of Dimes "Every Baby Has a Story" (www.everybabyhasastory.org)

March of Dimes (for NICU families)
(www.marchofdimes.com/prematurity/index_nicu.asp)

March of Dimes "Share Your Story" (www.shareyourstory.org)

Recommended Reading

Newborn Intensive Care: What Every Parent Needs to Know,
by Jeanette Zaichkin.

Parenting Your Premature Baby and Child: The Emotional Journey,
by Deborah L. Davis and Mara T. Stein.

Preemies: The Essential Guide for Parents of Premature Babies,
by Dana W. Linden, Emma T. Paroli, and Mia W. Doron.

The Preemie Parents' Companion: The Essential Guide to Caring for Your Premature Baby in the Hospital, at Home, and Through the First Years,
by Susan Madden.